SAFETY

SAFETY
Principles & Issues

Dean F. Miller
University of Toledo

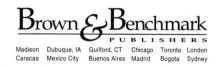

Madison   Dubuque, IA   Guilford, CT   Chicago   Toronto   London
Caracas   Mexico City   Buenos Aires   Madrid   Bogota   Sydney

Book Team

Editor *Edward Bartell*
Production Editor *Terry Routley*
Art Editor *Renee Grevas*
Visuals/Design Developmental Specialist *Janice Roerig-Blong*
Production Manager *Beth Kundert*
Visuals/Design Freelance Specialist *Mary L. Christianson*
Marketing Manager *Pamela S. Cooper*

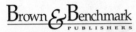

A Division of Wm. C. Brown Communications, Inc.

Executive Vice President/General Manager *Thomas E. Doran*
Vice President/Editor in Chief *Edgar J. Laube*
Vice President/Production *Vickie Putman*
National Sales Manager *Bob McLaughlin*

Wm. C. Brown Communications, Inc.

President and Chief Executive Officer *G. Franklin Lewis*
Senior Vice President, Operations *James H. Higby*
Corporate Senior Vice President and President of Manufacturing *Roger Meyer*
Corporate Senior Vice President and Chief Financial Officer *Robert Chesterman*

The credits section for this book begins on page 291 and is considered an extension of the copyright page.

Cover design by Kay Fulton Design

Cover images (top to bottom) © Cathlyn Melloan/Tony Stone Worldwide; Terry Vine/Tony Stone Images; Tom McCarthy/PhotoEdit

Photo research by Efrem Weitzman

Copyedited by Mary Agria

Copyright © 1995 by Wm. C. Brown Communications, Inc. All rights reserved

A Times Mirror Company

Library of Congress Catalog Card Number: 94–071726

ISBN 0–697–10943–7

No part of this publication may be reproduced, stored in a retrieval system, or transmitted, in any form or by any means, electronic, mechanical, photocopying, recording, or otherwise, without the prior written permission of the publisher.

Printed in the United States of America by Wm. C. Brown Communications, Inc., 2460 Kerper Boulevard, Dubuque, IA 52001

10 9 8 7 6 5 4 3 2 1

CONTENTS

Preface xiii

1 Injury—a Concern to All in Society 1

Introduction 1
Extent of the Problem 3
Defining the Terms 5
Causes of Unintentional Injury Events 6
   Human Factors 7
   Mechanical Factors 9
   Environmental Factors 10
Accident Repetition 10
Interactions and Relationships 13
Epidemiological Model Applied to Safety 16
   The Host 18
   The Etiological Agent—the Cause 19
   Environmental Factors 20
Health Objectives for the Nation—Unintentional Injuries 22
Summary 24
Discussion Questions 25
Suggested Readings 25
Endnotes 26

2 The Home—Injury Occurs in the Privacy of Where We Live 29

Introduction 29
At-Risk Age Groups 30
   Children 30
   The Elderly 31

Falls—a Major Injury Threat   32
Selected Danger Areas   34
   Kitchen   34
   Bathroom   35
   Television Set   36
   Fireplace   37
Specialized Power Tools and Equipment   38
   Home Workshops   38
   Chainsaws   39
   Lawnmowers   41
   Snow Throwers   42
Electricity   43
Flammable Liquids   46
Mobile Homes   48
Holiday Seasons   50
Summary   53
Discussion Questions   54
Suggested Readings   54
Endnotes   55

3   Consumer Safety—Careful Purchasing of Items for Household Use   57

The Consumer   57
The Consumer Product Safety Commission   59
   The Legislation   59
   Commission Activities   59
National Electronic Injury Surveillance System (NEISS)   62
Working Relationships Between CPSC and Other Agencies   62
Consumer Product Concerns   63
   Flammable Fabrics Act   63
   Fabric Flammability   63
   Consumer Product Labeling   65
Aerosols   66
Poisoning   67
   Causes of Poisoning   67
   Poison Prevention Packaging Act   70
   Impact of Regulation   70
   Aspirin Poisoning   71
   Poison Prevention Measures   72
   Poison Control Centers   73
Toy Safety   74
Summary   77
Discussion Questions   78
Suggested Readings   78
Endnotes   79

4 Fire—a Positive and a Negative Force 81

Introduction 81
What Is Fire? 82
Classifications of Fires 83
   Class A Fire 83
   Class B Fire 84
   Class C Fire 84
   Class D Fire 85
Data Regarding Fires 85
   Risk Factors 86
Types of Injuries Related to Fire 87
   Degree of Burn 88
   Scalding 88
   Other Fire-Related Hazards 88
   Medical Procedures for Burns 89
Early Warning Systems 90
   Types of Systems 90
   Location of the Systems 92
   Mandatory Regulations 92
Extinguishing Fires 92
   Portable Fire Extinguishers 93
   Community Fire-Fighting Systems 94
Fire Protection and Prevention 95
Summary 98
Discussion Questions 99
Suggested Readings 99
Endnotes 101

5 Safety in the Workplace—Economic as Well as Personal Concerns 103

Introduction 104
Workplace Safety Data 104
History of Occupational Safety 105
Occupational Safety and Health Act of 1970 109
   Purpose of the Legislation 110
   Areas of Mandated Activity 111
   Relationship of OSHA with the States 116
   Impact of OSHA 117
Occupational Safety Objectives for the Year 2000 119
Personnel Involved in Occupational Safety 121
   Industrial Hygienists 121
   Safety Engineers 121
   Occupational Physicians and Nurses 121
Selected Work Sites 122
   Mining 122
   Transportation 125

Employee Occupational Safety Initiatives   125
   Personal Protective Equipment   126
   Employee Motivational Programs   126
Summary   127
Discussion Questions   128
Suggested Readings   129
Endnotes   130

6   Rural Safety—Working and Living in the Rural Environment   133

Introduction   133
Injury in the Rural Setting   134
Government Regulation and Agriculture   136
Farm Machinery   137
   Risk Factors Associated with Farm Machinery   137
   Power-Driven Farm Machine Components   138
   Tractors   139
Grain Storage   143
   Fire   143
   Entrapment   144
   Lack of Ventilation   145
Exposure to Toxic Gases   145
Danger of Chemicals   146
Electrocution and Electrical Shock   148
Safety Concerns in Other Rural Occupations   149
Summary   150
Discussion Questions   151
Suggested Readings   151
Endnotes   152

7   The Motor Vehicle—Necessity and Potential Hazard   155

Introduction   155
Accident Statistics   157
Causes of Motor Vehicle Crashes   158
   Human Factors   158
   Age Factors   159
   Vehicular Factors   159
   Environmental Factors   160
Motor Vehicle Operation and Alcohol Use   162
   Physiology of Drinking   162
   Effects of Alcohol on Driving   163
   Driving Under the Influence   164
   Public Policy and Alcohol-Related Crashes   165
Motor Vehicle Collisions   170

　　　　Impact Restraints   171
　　　　　　Active Restraints—Seat Belts   171
　　　　　　Passive Restraints   175
　　　　Speed Limits   178
　　　　Pedestrian Safety   179
　　　　Safety at Rail Crossings   180
　　　　Summary   181
　　　　Discussion Questions   182
　　　　Suggested Readings   183
　　　　Endnotes   185

8　Forces of Nature—Cause of Many Fatalities and Injuries   189

　　　　Introduction   189
　　　　Tornadoes   190
　　　　Hurricanes   193
　　　　Lightning   197
　　　　Blizzards   199
　　　　Floods   201
　　　　Earthquakes   203
　　　　Summary   207
　　　　Discussion Questions   208
　　　　Suggested Readings   209
　　　　Endnotes   209

9　Recreational Pursuits—Leisure Time Activities and the Need for Safety   211

　　　　Introduction   211
　　　　Motorized Recreational Vehicles   213
　　　　　　Snowmobiles   213
　　　　　　Motorcycles   216
　　　　　　Minibikes   219
　　　　　　All-Terrain Vehicles (ATVs)   221
　　　　Outdoor Recreational Activities   222
　　　　　　Camping   222
　　　　　　Hunting   223
　　　　　　Skiing   225
　　　　Cycling   227
　　　　　　The Bicycle—a Toy or Not?   228
　　　　　　Cycle Construction and Operation   229
　　　　　　Personal Gear   229
　　　　　　Rules of the Road   230
　　　　Public Playgrounds   231
　　　　Summary   232
　　　　Discussion Questions   233

Suggested Readings   233
Endnotes   235

10 Water Safety   237

Introduction   237
Drowning   239
Swimming   240
   Open Bodies of Water   241
   Home Swimming Pools   241
   Community Swimming Pools   242
Boating   243
   Rules of the Water   244
   Specific Boating Safety Issues   245
   Handling Boat Capsizes   249
   Alcohol Consumption and Boating   249
   Nonmotorized Boating   250
Safety on the Ice   250
Other Water Activities   252
   Surfing   252
   Skin Diving   253
   Scuba Diving   253
   Water Skiing   255
Water Instruction Programs   255
Summary   256
Discussion Questions   256
Suggested Readings   257
Endnotes   258

11 School Safety—Impacting People from Preschool Through the Adult Years   259

Introduction   260
Safety as Part of the Total Curriculum   260
   Historical Foundations   260
Safety Instruction   261
   Correlation in Specific Contexts   262
   The Planned Safety Curriculum   264
   Curriculum Packages   265
   Preschool Safety Instruction   267
   Teaching to a Plan   267
   Content of Safety Curricula   268
Safe School Environment   268
   The School Playground   270
School Bus Transportation   270
   Seat Belts   272
   The Bus Driver   273

    Bus Maintenance   274
    Bus Routes   275
Emergency Care   275
School Accident Records   278
Emergency Drills   279
    Fire Drills   279
    Tornado Drills   280
Student Involvement   280
School Athletics   281
    Personal Equipment   282
    Facilities   282
    Supervision   283
    Medical Care   284
Summary   285
Discussion Questions   285
Suggested Readings   286
Endnotes   287

Glossary   289

Credits   291

Index   293

PREFACE

No one is immune from unintentional injury. Individuals of every gender, racial group, and age experience problems associated with injury-related circumstances. Such situations can result in minor injuries, disabling injuries, economic loss, psychological upheaval, and all too often death. The universality of unintentional injury increases the importance of safety programs and injury prevention initiatives.

An individual's attitude toward safety is affected by his or her knowledge, general attitudes, environment, and physical structure. One person will consciously work at injury prevention, while another will give little thought to actions that can prevent injury and death until a potentially hazardous situation arises.

Injury prevention and the practice of positive safety behavior is more than an individual concern. Because all people live in community, the dynamics of safety take on corporate dimensions. Many agencies and organizations have been established to assist an individual who becomes injured. Also, many of these community organizations carry out initiatives designed to foster a safer living and working environment.

However, beyond the unintentional injury statistics and the issue of community impact and response, there is also the human dimension. Any injury, disability, or fatality affects individual lives. Many of these individuals are people who never planned to become involved in a hazardous situation or gave much consideration to their personal safety behavioral patterns.

This book focuses on common areas of daily life—activities and situations in which people are likely to spend much of their waking hours. In each chapter various problems related to injury prevention and control are discussed. Hopefully, such an analysis will make readers more aware of conditions that can cause unintentional injury, and in turn, will prompt them to develop a safety consciousness in all aspects of their lives.

The first chapter presents an overview of the field of safety itself, including a number of general safety concepts that will underlie the entire book. Incorporated is up-to-date thinking of safety professionals regarding the most effective implementation strategies to create a safer world in which injury statistics can be reduced.

For many individuals, a significant amount of time is spent in a home environment. Chapters 2 and 3 focus upon home safety and consumer safety concerns. A variety of factors are examined that relate to unintentional injury and potential fatality in the home environment.

The content of chapter 4 is fire safety. Fire causes extensive loss, pain, and sorrow, not only in homes but in numerous other settings. Prevention is a major underlying concept that must be employed as one considers how to reduce loss related to fires.

Many efforts have been made to provide a safer working environment in business and industry. The Occupational Safety and Health Act (1970) was established to improve working conditions within the workplace. Information in chapter 5 examines a number of issues and concerns related to workplace safety and various public policy initiatives designed to make the workplace safer for all employees. In chapter 6, specific safety information is included relating to individuals who work in the rural, particularly the agricultural, environment.

The motor vehicle has revolutionized the world since its introduction in the latter part of the nineteenth century. Chapter 7 examines a number of considerations related to motor vehicle safety. A major emphasis of this chapter is on the role of public policy in working toward a safer community with fewer injuries and fatalities resulting from motor vehicle collisions.

Many unintentional injuries and fatalities occur as a result of acts of nature. Chapter 8 examines types of natural calamities that affect millions of people each year.

With increasing interest in recreational pursuits the potential for unintentional injury and fatality has expanded. Chapter 9 presents information about several selected recreational activities and considers measures that should be incorporated to make for a safer recreational setting. Many recreational pursuits occur on and around water. Drowning is a major cause of death for certain age groups. In chapter 10, a number of safety issues are raised in conjunction with boating, swimming, and other water-related recreational activities.

From preschool age through the adult years, most Americans spend a significant amount of time in some type of school environment. Chapter 11 discusses school safety. Instructional programs in safety education vary according to educational level and geographical setting. Initiatives need to be implemented in the schools to protect students from injury and to provide care should one become injured while at school. School safety must include a discussion of the role of injury prevention for participants in athletic programs. Measures need to be taken to reduce the number of injuries without decreasing the quality of athletic competition.

Safety is a dynamic field—constantly changing, presenting new challenges, and offering opportunities for creative thinking, research, and public policy initiatives. While a "zero" level of injury occurrence will never be possible, one must be hopeful that increased knowledge and awareness will lead to more positive safety behavioral patterns. Hopefully, everyone who reads this book will be more cognizant of the potential for a safer lifestyle, and in turn, will feel motivated to implement more positive safety behaviors in all aspects of life.

Special thanks to the reviewers who so graciously contributed to the work on this book:

Donald G. Carter
Western Kentucky University

Ronald L. Budig
Illinois State University

Ronald E. Puhl
Bloomsburg University, PA

D. F. M.

SAFETY

CHAPTER 1

Injury—a Concern to All in Society

Chapter Outline

Introduction
Extent of the Problem
Defining the Terms
Causes of Unintentional
   Injury Events
     Human Factors
     Mechanical Factors
     Environmental Factors
Accident Repetition
Interactions and Relationships
Epidemiological Model
   Applied to Safety
   The Host
   The Etiological Agent—
     the Cause
   Environmental Factors
Health Objectives for the
   Nation—Unintentional
   Injuries
Summary
Discussion Questions
Suggested Readings
Endnotes

Introduction

In terms of loss of life, disabling injury, interruption of daily activities and responsibilities, and economic costs, accidents take a heavy toll in American society. No one has escaped involvement in some type of injurious circumstance. It can be safely stated that every individual has had at least one, and probably several, injury-producing experiences.

    Some of these occurrences can be considered to be inconsequential. We bruise a knee in a fall; we stub a toe on the stairway; we cut ourselves with a small tool while working in the garage; or we bump our head and cut it as we get out of the automobile. Millions of such minor accident-related injuries never are reported. We probably do not even remember them several days after they happen. A physician is never contacted; the individual does not miss any classes at school or time from work; the injury is cared for individually; and friends or family do not even know that anything of consequence has taken place.

Throughout the course of our daily activities, each of us encounters situations which present the possibility of personal injury. Most people give little thought to the potential for injury in these everyday experiences. No doubt this is as it should be. If we let our constant exposure to an environment filled with potential injury worry us, we would become neurotic and nonfunctional. We might never carry out our normal daily activities. Certainly we would not consider driving our motor vehicles, and we probably would not function effectively at our place of employment. Even staying home would engender fear.

Nevertheless, it is necessary that an individual have a realistic view of life and the reality and likelihood of injury-producing circumstances. We all should strive toward improving our individual lifestyle in order to experience as safe an environment as possible.

Many people feel that accidents are likely to happen to someone else, rather than to them. We consider that if we are careful, have confidence in our ability to carry out certain skills and tasks, and remain alert, nothing of major consequence resulting in fatality and/or injury is likely to take place. However, this simply is not so. We must recognize our personal vulnerability to injury producing situations in every setting that we find ourselves and strive to develop attitudes and behaviors that will lessen the possibility of unintentional injury.

Some people regard accidents as a matter of statistical probability—the avoidance of a serious accidental occurrence is seen as "luck." Others respond to the possibility of having an accident that results in injury, loss of time from work, or necessitating medical attention by a kind of fatalism: "If it's my time, then there is nothing I can do about it" or "I'll have an accident if it's God's will." These and other such statements do not take into account the fact that one can, and must, take measures to protect against injury-causing situations.

It is important that each of us develop a safety consciousness that will result in positive behaviors as much as is possible. To do this we need to recognize both the reality of potential accidents and the role of attitude development and behavioral patterns in protecting against possible traumatic situations.

Many people think that the term *accidents* implies involvement with events that are not predictable—i.e., phenomenon over which we

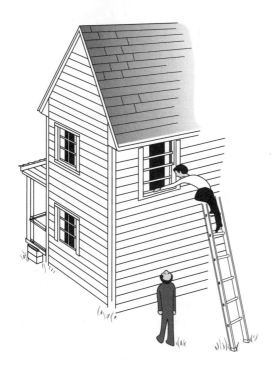

"Don't worry, I won't fall—I'm not prone to accidents, and furthermore it's not my time to have an accident!!"

have little control. This mind-set suggests that events resulting in injury or fatality cannot be predicted or prevented. It connotes the idea of chance. In fact, injury-causing situations can be prevented by taking appropriate actions, both individual and corporate.

Injury prevention needs to focus not only on individual factors, but it is a matter for community public policy initiatives. Safety program development and injury prevention and control initiatives should be the concern and emphasis of everyone.

Extent of the Problem

Unintentional injuries are the fifth leading cause of death in the United States, following heart disease, cancer, strokes, and bronchitis/emphysema.[1] Among school-aged children, adolescents, and young adults, accident-related injuries are the leading cause of death. During the high school and college years unintentional injuries are responsible for more fatalities than all other causes of death combined. Based on such statistics alone, it is imperative that the teenager and young adult learn to consider personal behavioral patterns as they relate to potentially hazardous and injury-producing situations.

Not only do thousands of fatalities occur each year but an estimated 3.4 million years of potential life are lost due to unintentional injury-producing circumstances.[2] This long-term productivity loss is greater than for the other four leading causes of death combined, primarily because so many injury-caused fatalities occur to people in their most productive years (the teens to the mid-40s). In addition to the many fatalities, nearly 17 million disabling injuries are reported annually.[3]

The economic costs of injury are a major concern to most people. A Congressional Report stated that the cost of injury in the United States exceeds $157 billion annually.[4] These costs involve medical expenditures, including the care, treatment, and rehabilitation of injured persons. Other economic factors related to injury-causing situations include wage losses resulting from the injury and property damage such as fire losses.

Statistics suggest that fatalities and injuries resulting from accidents occur on a scale comparable to that of a major national disaster. The National Safety Council places the number of annual deaths resulting from accidents at about 83,000.[5] The federal government in a major report on injury in America indicated that there are approximately 140,000 injury-related deaths per year.[6] One can only imagine the national concern and fear if an equal number of persons were to die in a twelve-month period from some communicable disease. Major media presentations, research initiatives, governmental actions, and increased funding would be targeted in an attempt to "solve" the problem. It must be asked why there is not the same concern relating to injury and accident fatality causation in the United States that we see when faced with an epidemic of some communicable disease? The measles epidemic of the early 1990s and the HIV/AIDS epidemic of the past decade reflect such instances around which major public concern and initiatives have been established.

In analyzing the multitude of data that exists, it is common to look at the statistics for specific categories of accident mortality. In doing so it becomes easy to overlook the human factor. Each statistical "count of one" is tragic in and of itself. It means not only that a number of potentially productive life-years has been lost, but that an important person—a parent, a son or daughter, a lover, husband or wife, or a friend—has ceased to live. A tragic void in someone's life has been created.

Defining the Terms

The term *safety* is used in several different contexts in our society, which can lead to confusion and misunderstanding. When talking about freedom from a communicable disease or some related health problem, we often say that we are "safe" from infection, such as when immunization has provided protection. To be "safe" means to be free from being able to get the disease. The term also has been widely used in discussing measures that can protect against getting AIDS—i.e., to practice "safe" sex.

The concept of safety also is used widely in the context of protecting personal belongings (such as a car, furniture, and other possessions) or one's person from external threats. For example, a person who lives in an apartment in a high-rise building in the city may desire to make sure that the building is "safe," meaning that there is a reasonable degree of protection for possessions and a lack of danger from personal attack or harm. Normally, this reference is not made with the thought of unintentional injury in mind. Rather, the concern is for premeditated external acts such as robbery. To be "safe" is to experience a degree of peace of mind regarding one's personal well-being.

Use of the term safety in relationship to events causing unintentional injury leads to the concept of accidents. An *accident* has been defined as an occurrence that disrupts the flow of normal interactions and relationships. These events usually produce unintended injury, death, or property damage.[7] Cause of such a disruption may be the result of the action or inaction of individuals; the action of animals (as when Mrs. O'Leary's cow kicked over a lantern in Chicago, causing much destruction from fire); or the action of nature (natural forces such as tornadoes, hurricanes, floods, and lightning).

The National Research Council of the National Academy of Science in 1966 identified accidental death and disability as the neglected disease of modern society. Since that time, there have been various calls by health and safety agencies, governmental commissions, and other respected safety and law enforcement organizations for increased initiatives to correct, improve, and modify injury-producing situations. As a result, injury causation and prevention have become identified as a major public health and community concern in America. Various public health strategies have been designed to reduce injury-causing circumstances with particular emphasis on the need for multidisciplinary efforts in program development, education, research, and other initiatives.

In 1987 a major conference on injury in America was held after which a number of important recommendations were published that have had significant impact.[8] The conference report suggests that to promote better public understanding and program support, the word "accident" should be eliminated and use of the concept of injury should become the norm.[9] *Injury* is identified as "unintentional or intentional damage to the body resulting from acute exposure to thermal, mechanical, electrical, or chemical energy or from the absence of such essentials as heat or oxygen."[10] In short, a major outcome of the 1987 conference report was to shift public focus from the concept of accident prevention—which is misunderstood by many people to mean they have no control over circumstances resulting in injuries—to the issue of injury prevention and control, factors we can more readily understand, study, and prevent.

Among the further recommendations of this conference was the call for the creation of a federal agency to focus financial and research resources on the problem. As a result, the Center for Environmental Health and Injury Control was established as one of the operating centers that comprise the governmental Centers for Disease Control and Prevention (CDC). Research is supported by this agency with the goal of improving the safety of Americans in all settings: at work, in the home, on the highways, in recreational pursuits, and in numerous other settings. A major program responsibility of this governmental agency is increasing the public's awareness of injuries, particularly injury prevention, through educational initiatives.

Thinking, discussions, and recommendations coming out of the 1987 Conference on Injury in America have led to a better understanding and agreement regarding the concept of what constitutes "safety." This agreement among many agencies and organizations—governmental, private sector, law enforcement, and educational—makes for clearer program development, funding initiatives, and organizational cooperation.

Causes of Unintentional Injury Events

When considering matters relating to injury prevention, it is necessary to examine the various causes of unintentional injury events. Usually there is no one single factor that can be identified as the sole cause of

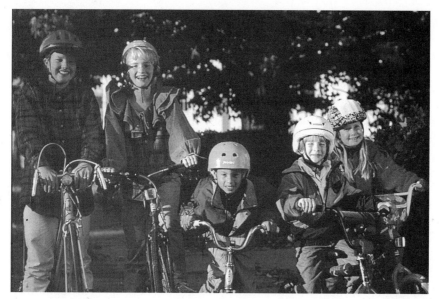

Development of motor skills involved in riding a bicycle are necessary to reduce the possibility of a young child being injured. Skill development should begin at a very early age.

a specific unintentional injury event. Rather, there are numerous interrelated factors involved. These may be identified as human factors, mechanical factors, and environmental factors.

Human Factors

Often the primary causes of an injury resulting circumstance center upon the individual or *human factors*. What did the individual do that led to the situation? What do we know about the individual's attitude that resulted in the injury-causing event? Did the child have adequate skills to operate the tractor, snowmobile, or boat that was involved in the situation?

Very often the degree of individual skill involved in operating the machine, equipment, or vehicle is a major consideration. People will perform psychomotor skills successfully within the limits of their own individual training, experience, and abilities. Failure to operate within one's motor skill limits can cause a serious injury-producing situation to occur. For example, the young child who has not developed the skills required to ride a bicycle is more likely to experience an injury-resulting situation than is the person who has developed specific bicycle-riding skills. The youngster performing on a piece of gymnastic equipment without well-developed skills is more likely to lose balance, fall, and sustain injuries than is the more experienced, skilled performer. The more experience the employee has in operating a complex piece of machinery, the more skillful will be the performance and the less likely it is that an injury will occur. This principle is true of most skills involving physical motor activities.

The presence of a positive attitude regarding safety is another factor impacting injury-resulting situations. For many people, safety and injury prevention basically focuses on adhering to certain rules and regulations. This attitude begins in early childhood when children are instructed not to touch the stove or not to place a pencil in the electrical outlet. Thus, children come to relate safe practices to obeying or following the instructions of their parents or other adults. For adults at work, listings of rules and regulations to be followed are posted in the workplace. The employee is expected to obey these policies, often without understanding the rationale or reason for them.

However, an attitude of safety consciousness needs to go beyond such external focus on rules to recognizing the necessity for regulatory enforcement. It takes the establishment of positive attitudes to lead to behavior patterns that promote positive safety practices. All the regulations and rules that one can list are of little value if one's attitudes regarding adherence to them are negative. This can be seen in situations where individuals do not adhere to speed limits, as a result of an attitude that the speed limit does not personally apply or that the limit is unrealistic considering the circumstances (hence there is no reason to reduce one's speed).

Motivating the general public, particularly young people, to develop positive attitudes toward safety practices is not always easy. Many teenagers and young adults do not feel that they are vulnerable to circumstances that can cause serious injury or death. This likelihood often is the farthest thing from their minds—an attitude which can result in a serious, even fatal, incident.

Not to be overlooked when considering the causes of accidents in society are individual physiological impairments, such as vision, hearing, and reaction time. Physical impairment may be the result of natural physiological processes. This is noted particularly as one becomes older. The senior citizen must learn to accommodate to changes in hearing or visual acuity and to reduced motor abilities; reaction time tends to become lengthened and balance may be less steady. Such impairments, regardless of age, demand adaptation and modification of individual practices. At the other extreme, excessive reliance on physiological capabilities—e.g., exceptional reflexes in athletes or young adults—may impair judgment in specific situations where more caution is warranted.

Many substances have detrimental effects upon the physical performance of an individual. Most commonly considered is the effect of abuse substances of alcohol and drugs. Statistics point out that as many as one-half of all motor vehicle fatalities and a majority of boating fatalities, along with hundreds of hours of lost work time and numerous other injury-related losses, involve alcohol use and intoxication. It is understandable why there is increased concern by the public and media, as well as researchers for substance abuse issues.

There also has been interest in the role of emotion as a cause of unintentional injury events. Emotions such as anger, hostility, rebellion, and frustration may lead to recklessness which in turn can result in injury-causing events. Inattention to tasks such as operation of a snow blower, riding a lawn tractor, operation of a motor vehicle, use of a chain saw, or other piece of farm, home, or industrial equipment for as brief a time as a single second may create conditions that lead to serious injury or fatality.

Particular equipment itself may induce emotions that lead to accidents. Some psychologists suggest that this may be so. For example, the power at one's command operating a motor vehicle may serve as a substitute for something that the individual feels is lacking in one's own personality. If an individual has a sense of inferiority or a lack of self-esteem, as soon as the power and weight of the motor vehicle is at that person's command, attitudes and feelings may be released which overcompensate—resulting all too often in serious problems of judgment that can have dangerous, even fatal results.

It has also been suggested that accidents and their accompanying injuries may even help resolve certain emotional needs of some people. Having an accident is not considered by most people to be an antisocial behavior—the possible exception being drunk driving; yet an accident may bring attention to an individual that might not be otherwise forthcoming. Witness what happens if you go to class or to work with your leg in a cast or your forehead bandaged. Normally, people inquire about what happened and how you are feeling. More interest will be shown by your colleagues than is the case on a routine work day, and numerous statements of concern, expressions of sorrow about your condition, and sympathy will likely be expressed.

Mechanical Factors

Not all injury-producing circumstances are the sole result of human failure. Many times we focus our educational efforts, our remedial initiatives, and our accident investigations only upon the actions of the individual. Yet many fatal and injury-resulting situations occur from some kind of *mechanical failure*. The breakdown may be something rather mild, as when some part of the bicycle fails to function properly resulting in injury to the rider. On the other hand, mechanical failure can lead to tragedies causing hundreds of deaths, as when there is an engine failure in an airplane.

As careful and precise as manufacturers of products try to be, there is always the possibility of mechanical failure. There are many measures that can be taken to reduce risk due to such failures. Improved engineering, manufacturing, and quality control strategies can reduce the possibility of mechanical failure. Also, regular maintenance of engines and mechanical parts that involve movement and friction or wear must be considered a major preventive measure that will help to reduce the risk of unintentional injury events.

An increasing awareness of mechanical failures has developed in the field of motor vehicle safety and in the consumer product safety movement. There have been numerous product and vehicle recalls by the manufacturers as they become aware of potentially dangerous products. Sometimes these recalls involve complete removal of the product from the marketplace. In other instances the manufacturer will replace the part that is the cause of the possible danger.

Environmental Factors

Innumerable factors in our surroundings, so-called *environmental factors*, may contribute to unintentional injury events. In the case of motor vehicle operation, the roadway conditions are of principal concern. Throughout the months of the year roadway conditions vary in many parts of the country. For example, a rainfall will cause a wet surface that easily may cause one to lose control of the motor vehicle. Snow, sleet, and ice are other natural occurrences that cause many accidents. The design and construction of the roadway introduces many other factors that may contribute to possible vehicle collisions.

Within the workplace there are many conditions that can be primary causes of injuries. There may be substances on the floor that can cause an injury. The presence and proximity of high-speed equipment that is used daily at the factory may create an environment conducive to injury, and possible fatality.

Accident Repetition

If one were to take a cross-section of any population group, as is presented in the Issue—Case Study exercise, a majority of those surveyed have never been involved in an accident requiring medical attention.

> **A CASE STUDY APPROACH TO ISSUES**
> **Surveys of Accident Repetition**
>
> Conduct a survey of any group of people asking how many have never had a broken bone. In all probability close to seventy-five percent of the group will so identify themselves. Then ask the remainder, those who have had at least one fracture, to stand. Somewhere close to one-fourth of the class or group will be standing. Ask those who have had only one fracture to sit down. Then ask those still standing how many fractures they have had. Typically, the greatest number of fractures have occurred to a small portion of the group members. (Note: in this survey we are suggesting that having a fracture was *not* a planned event, but rather an unintentional injury.)
>
> What might we learn as we analyze this small percentage of people who have experienced a high number of accidental fractures? What are some of the factors associated with circumstances resulting in their fractures? Do these people tend to have an unusually large number of other accidental situations?
>
> There are many things that can be learned about the accident repeater from this type of survey. Such issues are of concern to many involved in safety programs in a variety of settings.

Most employees never are injured on the job. A small minority of those polled would account for a vast majority of all injuries. Anyone who has taught school-age children will have noticed this fact. Most children never get hurt or become injured while at school. It is the same few who are continually being injured, who cut themselves, fall and break an arm, or are hurt while playing on the playground equipment or in the gymnasium so that they require services of the school nurse. Not only is it a relatively few who are injured, but inevitably these few seem to experience more than one or two injury situations each school year.

What are we to conclude from these observations? Do accidents occur basically to a selected group of people? If so, are there certain emotional, psychological, physiological, and/or personality characteristics that are common to those individuals who are accident repeaters?

Accident repetition has both financial and legal repercussions. Employees who tend to be involved in excessive numbers of accidents at the worksite are of particular concern to the corporate management. Another obvious concern is the accident repeater who has several insurance claims resulting from motor-vehicle collisions. It takes very few such claims for the insurance carrier to cancel the coverage. Laws and penalties for drunk driving are much more stringent for the person who has had numerous citations.

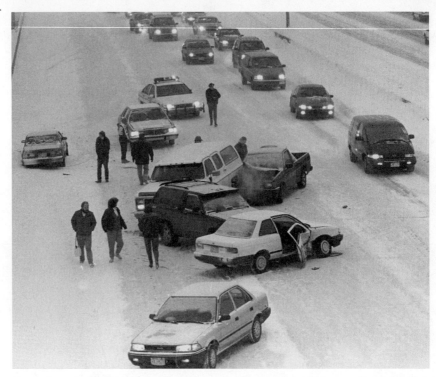

Natural occurrences involving snow, ice, and sleet may result in many injury and fatality producing collisions.

For many years it was assumed that there was such a thing as an accident-prone personality—that multiple accidents were associated with certain personality characteristics. These characteristics, it was suggested, led to a tendency to become involved in various unsafe behaviors. Individuals with an abnormal number of accidents were assumed to have certain identifiable traits. As a result, researchers tried to identify specific traits that could indicate likely candidates for injury-induced behavior. It was suggested that as we learn more about the particular traits of accident repeaters, steps might be taken to reduce the incidence of fatal and injury-producing events.

Today, this thinking has been largely discounted. The concept of the accident-prone personality began to be questioned in the early 1960s, particularly by a number of American psychologists.[11] Since that time, many safety scientists and psychologists have repudiated the notion of an accident-prone personality. They suggest that there is no definite proof or identification of specific emotional, psychological, physiological, or personality traits that could differentiate the accident repeater from that individual who has had few or no accidents.

Many of the conclusions regarding accident proclivity were formulated from study in one field of accident causation, motor-vehicle safety. These findings were then applied to other kinds of activities and conditions. Because circumstances varied, it was doubtful that this practice of taking data from one area of safety and making general applications based on it was appropriate.

However, we cannot ignore the fact that certain people do experience an abnormal number of unintentional injury events. Other health and safety fields legitimately focus attention and concern on such individuals who habitually are subject to specific debilitating conditions. For example, the person who comes down with a certain disease several different times would warrant concern from family, the physician, and even the public health authorities. Special care and treatment would be sought to help this person. It only seems logical to suggest that we need to be aware of factors which appear to be common among accident repeaters, although we should not conclude based on such patterns that safety programming and injury reduction initiatives need to be focused primarily on these individuals.

Injury prevention must examine and work toward improving and resolving this broader scope of injury and its causes. This, in part, calls for increased research into the relationship between environmental and personal factors in injury-prevention behavior. An emphasis upon individual behavior also suggests work with alternative strategies such as behavior modification. In addition, more needs to be learned about various kinds of positive incentives that result in injury prevention. The role of safety education as a primary preventive measure cannot be overlooked.

Interactions and Relationships

Major safety programming and research today tend to center on the interactions and relationships between an individual, the environment, and human behavioral patterns. The result is increased study of educational interventions that can impact human safety behavioral practices and of measures that can be taken to provide for a safer environment.

Safety promotion strategies—especially activities directed toward positive individual actions and behavioral change—have been of growing interest in the past several years in the fields of health and safety. The purpose of effective safety instructional initiatives is to bring about positive behavioral patterns, be it the study of fire prevention measures, an industrial lesson on machine and equipment safety, a "DUI" class for persons convicted of driving while under the influence of alcohol, or a parent's explanation to a small child about the importance and necessity of not leaving toys on the stairs.

Research is being carried out to ascertain why people act as they do in matters related to injury prevention. Why do some people take chances that result in greater likelihood of accident? Why is there a dichotomy between knowledge and practice in fatality- and injury-causing situations? What attitudes encourage the use of protective equipment (e.g., wearing helmets when riding bicycles and motorcycles) and/or lead to the refusal to use such protective measures? This is just a small sample of the many questions in need of study, research, and discussion focused on obtaining greater knowledge about individual safety practices.

Much also needs to be learned about what teaching strategies are the most effective in bringing about the desired safety behaviors for a particular population group. A procedure useful among teenage boys may be totally ineffective for older adults or senior citizens. A movie presenting "gory" injury scenes may be useful for certain individuals, whereas others may simply hide their faces when confronted with these scenes on the movie or video screen. For the latter, the film may be only an endurance test to see if one is able to make it through the entire showing without becoming nauseous. The educational intent of the presentation becomes lost for these individuals.

Research efforts to learn more about what teaching methods and communication skills are most effective in safety instruction is necessary. As in all good teaching, instructors cannot simply present cognitive material (facts, figures, statistics, and safety lists) and automatically expect the result to be the establishment of positive safety attitudes that lead to effective safe practices. Student attitudes, value systems, backgrounds, and skill development must not be overlooked in developing safety instructional initiatives.

A number of behavior modification strategies have been used to improve the safety environment for a variety of groups. The emphasis has been to encourage positive reinforcement strategies rather than punishment. Positive reinforcement measures seem to be more beneficial in that they tend to increase self-esteem, whereas the use of fear and penalties tend to have a more negative impact on individuals. There is little evidence that the use of disciplinary penalties to improve safety are effective, particularly in occupational safety research.[12]

Many different incentives have been used to encourage the development of positive safety behaviors.[13] For example, monetary incentives have been used, particularly in the occupational setting. When an individual or industrial department goes a certain length of time without an injury-producing situation, various monetary awards are provided to the employees. Also, team competition has been used to encourage the practice of safe behaviors. Assertiveness training strategies and social reinforcement are other initiatives that have been successful in safety behavioral programs.

Research has shown that in the short term, incentives enhance safety performance and reduce accidents.[14] For example, studies show that individual reward has proven successful in promoting seat belt use. However, more information and data is needed in order to learn which types of incentives are most effective in encouraging other safety practices. Also in spite of the fact that safety education seems to lead to behavior change in specific areas, there is little evidence that such instructional measures have carry-over effect into other settings.

Preventive measures may need to be directed at not just modification of the behavior of an individual, but also at modifications in the environment. This often requires public policy changes, such as modifications in laws, ordinances, and regulations—not easy tasks to accomplish. For example, placing restrictions on the use of handguns, requiring the presence of passive restraints in all motor vehicles, or modification of vehicle design to reduce the possibility of fires following collisions are examples of measures that some have proposed to bring about change through the public policy arena. Such attempts have met with varying degrees of success in recent years.

Numerous laws have been passed designed to reduce unintentional injury events. Regulations, ordinances, and other guidelines abound (at local, state, and federal levels) that govern various safety-related contexts. For example, federal legislation calls for the establishment of performance standards in such diverse manufacturing areas as automobiles, poisonous product containers, and children's toys.

With thousands of laws, standards, and regulations written by so many different governmental agencies, various measures must be taken to assure compliance. Enforcement may be accomplished through the activities of the local law enforcement departments, whose responsibility it is to make sure that speed limits are obeyed and that motorists drive their vehicles in a safe manner. Licensing for the operation of a motorcycle or for fishing or hunting involve other enforcement agencies.

Enforcement procedures also include investigatory programs to ascertain whether required industrial safety measures are being adhered to for the safety of employees. These investigations are usually carried out by OSHA (Occupational Safety and Health Administration) compliance officers.

Enforcement measures may range from parental reminders when a child fails to obey a home safety regulation to imprisonment for arrest while driving under the influence of alcohol. Fines are a common enforcement deterrent. When a company fails to comply with certain occupational safety regulations, a fine will be levied. Driving a motor vehicle above the maximum speed limits can result in the issuing of a fine, and if a repeat offense, can lead to loss of driving privileges.

Safety enforcement measures are not simply focused on individual persons, but also are important in assuring that appropriate safety engineering measures have been taken in the design and construction processes of such things as motor vehicles, consumer products, roadways, buildings, and so on.

Numerous ordinances and regulations have been developed to provide protection from injury and death. Measures have been implemented to make vehicles and highways safer. Responsibility for providing a safe environment falls to some degree upon improved engineering and production techniques. The automotive engineer, the highway designer, the building architect, or the toy manufacturer all play important roles—that is, the provision of a safe environment relies upon the professional functions of many different kinds of design engineers.

The field of safety engineering is very broad. It involves the development of new designs and products as well as on various architectural activities focusing upon improved safety features in the construction of a building or any other kind of facility. For example, placement of handrails along stairs or the removal of dangerous objects in hallways reflect the work of building architects.

On the other hand, private individuals also can become involved on a personal basis in injury prevention. The public can request and demand the design of better quality and functional nonflammable children's clothing. They can expect their motor vehicles to be designed with safety in mind. Materials used in the construction of buildings should be strong and fire resistant; the manufacture of industrial safety equipment should provide protection to the human body.

Epidemiological Model Applied to Safety

The use of descriptive studies to trace the extent and distribution of unintentional injury events in a given population involves the application of the *epidemiological model.* Historically, the application of this model has been used principally in the field of communicable disease control. Epidemiology makes it possible to learn what the causative agents of a certain disease are and provides information about groups of individuals who are most likely to contract that specific disease. It has also been valuable in ascertaining the relationships between various illnesses and behavior patterns. Specific etiologies (causes) of diseases have been identified using the principles of epidemiology.

There are three interactive dimensions in the epidemiological model: a *host,* an *etiological agent,* and the *environment.* In order to control a communicable disease one needs to break the interactive chain of infection existing between these factors. Focus upon the individual—or host—involves studying those factors directed toward the person. It is the individual who is susceptible to the specific disease in a communicable disease control program. In communicable disease control it is the etiological agent, the specific microorganism, that causes the host to become ill. It is necessary for the agent to invade the host before a disease can become manifested in an individual.

The microorganism can invade the host through a number of avenues. These factors are spoken of as the environment. Some diseases are transmitted through airborne particles, others in water, insects carry many different microorganisms, and others are transmitted by direct person-to-person contact. As long as the host, the etiologic agent, and the environment are kept in equilibrium, a person is healthy. A maldisturbance leads to sickness. In disease control activities it is important to ascertain which dimension can be countered most easily, economically, and effectively in order to break the chain of infection.

The epidemiological model was first suggested in 1948 as an approach that could be used for the study and prevention of accidents.[15] The Kellogg Foundation funded several community-based safety projects in the 1950s using the host-agent-environment interactive epidemiology model. Since that time the model has been used extensively by researchers and programmers in the field of safety in many different settings.

The application of epidemiological methodology in injury causation and prevention has been found to be useful in identifying the causes of unintentional injury events. However, it must be noted that this model has its shortcomings. In communicable disease control work there usually is one single causative agent, such as a particular virus, bacterium, or protozoan. When the epidemiological model is applied to the field of safety, the approach becomes more problematical in that there usually is not one single causative agent. Unintentional injury events tend to be multicausal—causes which often involve a variety of different interactions, some nearly impossible to ascertain or pinpoint.

Analyzing the three factors of the epidemiological model will help clarify some of the issues involved.

The Host

The study of an unintentional injury event requires that the person, or persons, involved be the focus of study. This may mean the study of a specific population, as in the case of a study of farmers who are injured from working with high-speed farm machinery. It could be a study of the behavioral patterns of boys on the playground who are injured during a specific period of time and who require the services of the school nurse. Another example of the application of this model might be an examination of the physiological factors associated with falls resulting in hospitalization among senior citizens above the age of seventy.

After study is conducted to learn more about the various factors associated with the individual (the host) and the problem under consideration, it becomes important to apply the model to establishing an injury-reduction initiative. Since we are dealing with the host, our attention and program activities will focus upon the people involved. Injuries occur to people, not to inanimate objects. Numerous host-related factors are important in injury-causing situations, although two that usually receive a lot of notice are age and gender.

The age of an individual is related to the probability of being involved in an unintentional injury event. For example, there is significant data that shows that it is more likely for a male under the age of thirty to be involved in a motor vehicle collision than it is for an individual who is over forty. On the other hand, there is statistical evidence that the highest rate of unintentional fatalities occurs among the elderly, individuals over sixty-five years of age. Among the elderly, falls are the leading cause of unintentional death. The older the person, the more susceptible one is to falling and a resultant fatality.

Another important human (host) factor associated with injury is the gender of an individual. It is known that males have more unintentional injuries than females. More than two out of every three unintentional fatalities occur to males. A number of reasons have been identified for such a pattern. One is that males tend to be involved more often than women in activities that are potentially hazardous. For example, males account for nearly 90 percent of the fatalities and injuries associated with motorcycle collisions.

In establishing an injury prevention program, several activities can be conducted to make the person (host) less likely to have an unintentional injury. For example, the role of education and skill development are primary program emphases. As individuals better understand the danger of a particular situation and have increased

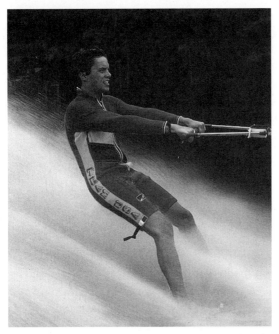

Hours of instruction and practice are needed before a person has developed the appropriate skills to barefoot waterski safely without injury. This is the case in all human practices requiring specific skills.

knowledge about how to protect against injury and fatality, there is the expectation of reduction of unintentional injury events.

Skill development is another important program focus. For example, the development of swimming or cycling skills play important roles in helping to reduce the likelihood of an injury situation. This is true of children as well as adults. As children develop physical coordination and basic skills in handling and playing with their toys there is a reduced likelihood of an injury occurring. Adults also have a reduced chance of injury if they learn how to safely handle and operate a power tool in the work area or in the yard. Regardless of the age or gender of an individual, skill development can help reduce the possibility of injury or fatality.

The Etiological Agent—the Cause

As we continue to apply the epidemiological model to injury prevention, we need to focus upon the causative agent. Many substances, products, and items may cause injury or death. The specific product may be of a chemical or biological nature that is systemically toxic to the host. This is the case when dealing with the many different kinds of household poisons, insecticides, pesticides, and herbicides that are usually found around homes, garages, and farm buildings.

On the other hand, the causative agent may inflict external damage, as with a piece of metal that flies into a person's eye while running a high-speed piece of machinery in the factory or a piece of wood that falls on the shoulder of the carpenter working on a new building. In the home, the causative agent could be a knife resting in the drawer that cuts a finger when one reaches in to retrieve something or flames from the grill over which an individual is preparing a steak for dinner that may cause a burn.

Any type of epidemiological study requires a careful analysis of the actual agent that caused the fatality or injury. Measures should be taken to reduce the presence of causative agents that can harm individuals. This could mean placing sharp tools in their proper storage places in the workplace when they are not in use. It might involve removing a child's toys and other objects from the stairways. Such a focus could mean purchasing a car, a riding lawn mower, or other types of power tools that have appropriate safety features installed.

Environmental Factors

In any given unintentional injury event there are a number of factors associated with environment that can be investigated. For example, during a serious windstorm a tree may fall on the car and cause injury to the occupant. The host is the individual who ventured out despite travelers' advisories; the agent of injury is the tree; and the environmental factor involved is a natural force, the wind.

Around any building—a home, office, school, or public building—various construction features of the structure could be the cause of injury. Possibly the simplest example would be a slippery floor, because of which an individual may slip and break an arm or hit one's head. The injury results from the environmental factor in the situation, the slippery floor. Similar is the case of an elderly person who slips while in the bathtub and is injured. The environmental factor associated with the injury is the type of surface on the bottom of the tub.

Many measures may be employed to reduce the hazardous nature of a given environment. In the case of highway safety, periodic engineering developments have made for safer travel, such as the use of breakaway sign poles and the construction of dual highways.

APPLICATION OF THE EPIDEMIOLOGICAL MODEL
Water Safety Programs to Reduce Drownings

Reduction of drowning provides a good example in which the epidemiological model can be applied. The office of injury control of the state health department has determined, upon examination of injury and fatality data, that there is a serious need to employ some type of programming initiatives to reduce drownings within the state. Where would be the best place to focus the resources of the department in this initiative?

The objective, to design a water safety/drowning prevention program, suggests that the three factors of the epidemiological model—the host, causative agent, and environmental relationships—be examined. A researcher must determine which of these three factors deserves the principle focus. Maybe actions could be directed toward all three. On the other hand, this might not be logical or possible.

Activities focusing specifically upon the host or the individuals involved could be directed toward providing instruction in swimming skills. The more skillful one is in swimming the less the risk of drowning. Education also can be provided in various other factors associated with drowning. Another initiative could be to make people more aware of the importance of supervision around pools, lakes, and other places where people swim. Knowing how to provide assistance to swimmers in trouble in the water is important. As in most injury prevention programs, education is an important dimension of such a host-related epidemiological model.

The causative agent associated with drowning situations is water. One can drown in any depth of water. However, because it is impossible to swim, to bathe, or participate in other aquatic activities without water, there is little that the safety programmer can do to eliminate the agent in a water safety program.

Much can be accomplished related to the environment in a water safety/drowning prevention program. Many measures relating to the construction of an outdoor pool should be taken into account. All outdoor pools should be fenced in to assure that people, particularly young children, will not enter the pool unsupervised. In many communities regulations have been established that are designed to protect against drowning and injury associated with home outdoor pools.

Drowning occurs in quiet ponds, in dangerous bodies of water, as well as at public beaches. After study of the location where drownings occur the department could institute measures to remove the dangers associated with these locations or draining of ponds might be a worthwhile action. Further analysis of data and examination of the particular situations should suggest other measures to control environmental factors relating to drowning.

It would seem, upon study and analysis, that in developing a water safety/drowning prevention program using the epidemiology model, the greatest effort should be centered on control of environmental factors and matters directed toward the host. Little, if anything, can be done concerning the causative agent.

Health Objectives for the Nation—Unintentional Injuries

In 1979, after reviewing data concerning the leading causes of death and/or morbidity in the United States, the federal government identified a number of specific risk factors related to the leading causes of death. In an effort to apply these data and work toward an improvement in individual lifestyles of the American citizen, five national health-related goals were established.

Following identification of these national goals, extensive professional review took place for the purpose of setting specific, measurable objectives to be obtained during the decade of the 1980s. These objectives were to serve as a focus and provide guidelines for health and safety organizations in the establishment of programs and for funding support—including federal agencies, state and local health departments, private businesses and industries, schools, safety organizations, and various health and safety community coalitions involved in programming directed at improving the well-being of the American public.

Eight of the objectives identified in 1979 focused upon accident prevention and injury control:

- Three centered upon the importance of risk reduction initiatives (increasing the number of automobiles with automatic restraint protection, ensuring that newborns return home after birth in certified passenger carriers, and requiring the installation of smoke alarm systems in homes and apartments.
- Two were designed to encourage and expand public and professional awareness of safety measures.
- One stated that parents should be able to identify appropriate measures to protect children from three major risks of injury, including motor-vehicle injuries, burns, and poisonings.
- Another objective called for health care providers to advise patients about the value of safety belts in automobiles.

Efforts to meet the identified objectives by 1990 met with mixed results. Some objectives were met, others were not. Nonetheless, the national health objectives initiative was expanded in 1990 with the publication of new objectives to be achieved by the year 2000.[16] (See Table 1.1.) Nearly 300 specific measurable objectives were identified and catalogued into 22 priority areas. One of these priority areas is unintentional injuries.[17] Within this category 22 specific objectives have been identified.

TABLE 1.1 Health Objectives to Be Achieved by the Year 2000—Fatalities

Type of Fatality	2000	Baseline Data (1989)
All unintentional injuries	29.3[1]	34.5
Motor vehicle crashes	1.9[2]	2.4
Falls and fall-related injuries	2.3	2.7
Drowning	1.3	2.1

[1]per 100,000 population
[2]per 100 million vehicle miles
Source: Department of Health and Human Services, *Healthy People 2000: National Health Promotion and Disease Prevention Objectives*, 1991.

One objective calls for the reduction of deaths caused by unintentional injuries as well as nonfatal unintentional injuries requiring hospitalization. Specific objectives suggest that by the year 2000 there should be a reduction of fatalities caused by motor vehicle crashes, falls, drownings, and fires. Objectives for reduction in nonfatal poisoning, serious head injuries, spinal cord and hip injuries were also included. Other objectives to be achieved by the year 2000 include reduction of alcohol use in injury causing circumstances, increased use of seat belts by occupants of motor vehicles, increased use of helmets by the riders of motorcycles and bicycles, and the presence of smoke detectors in homes and apartments.

In order to provide better education concerning injury prevention, the health objectives initiative called for increased provision of instruction on injury prevention and control as part of the school curriculum in all grades, kindergarten through grade 12. Also, measures should be expanded by primary health care providers to deliver counseling on safety precautions to prevent unintentional injury.

To achieve these objectives designed to reduce fatalities and unintentional injuries by the year 2000, all types of safety-related agencies and organizations must be aware of the initiative and inform their constituencies. This initiative will provide direction not only for programming, but also for research, establishment of public policy rules and regulations, as well as for special fund-raising activities.

Particular programming must be focused upon those high risk populations for each category. For example, children under the age of four, adults over 65, and African-American males and females are special population target groups identified to be at risk for experiencing death from residential fires. At special risk for death from drowning are young children, males between the ages of 15 and 34, and African-American males.

Summary

The concept of what constitutes safety may have different meanings for each person. Basically the focus in this chapter is upon those measures designed to prevent, or at least reduce, fatalities and injuries, resulting from sudden, unplanned, unintentional injury events.

Historically, in the field of safety, the term *accident* has been used by most people. The use of this term leads to the idea that fatalities and injuries are caused by random events that cannot be predicted or prevented. It suggests that there is little one can do to prevent an accident. In recent years there has been increasing focus on the concept of injury prevention. This concept of safety focuses the energies of individuals, as well as community agencies, upon the reduction of causative factors associated with unintentional injuries, risk factors, and design of effective preventive initiatives.

Every person experiences many different types of injuries throughout a lifetime. A broad range of causes of injury producing circumstances has been identified through research, analysis of data, and other sources of information. Some of these causes center around human factors, others are related to the manufacture, construction, and/or mechanical nature of items with which people come into contact. Also, the role of the environment can have an impact upon injury causation.

A large number of injuries occur to a relatively small number of individuals. This problem of the accident repeater is a matter of concern to business and industry, to the insurance business, as well as to others. At one time the idea was quite widely accepted that there was an accident-prone personality and that certain psychological and physiological characteristics associated with these persons could be identified. Today, the concept of the accident-prone personality is not widely accepted. However, concern about those individuals who repeatedly experience injury-producing circumstances continues.

The epidemiological model used in much public health and medical research has been applied to the field of safety prevention. This model involves the application of measures directed at either the host, the causative agent, or the environment—for the purpose of reducing the potential of an unintentional injury event.

The enormity of the problems associated with fatality and injury has been noted by the federal government. Hence, injury prevention is one of the priority areas identified in the health promotion and disease prevention objectives initiative. A number of measurable objectives have been identified for reducing unintentional injury by the year 2000.

Discussion Questions

1. Discuss the concepts related to the terms: *accident, safety,* and *injury prevention.*
2. What does the term *safety* mean to you?
3. What conclusions do you draw as you examine statistical data relating to fatalities and injuries?
4. What are some personal factors associated with unintentional injury events?
5. Explain the role of emotions in the cause of unintentional injury.
6. Do you feel that a focus upon accident repetition should be an area of primary emphasis in safety research and programming? Explain in detail the reasons for your answer.
7. Identify some of the ways in which law enforcement and legislation impact injury prevention programming.
8. How is the epidemiological model applied to injury prevention and control activities?
9. Give an example of an injury-producing situation and apply the epidemiological model to reducing the risks associated with the problem.
10. What are the significant objectives as identified by the federal government in the Health Objectives for the Nation, Year 2000 relating to unintentional injury?

Suggested Readings

"1987 Conference on Injury in America: A Summary." *Public Health Reports* 102, no. 6 (November–December 1987): 577–81.

Centers for Disease Control. "Cost of Injury—United States: A Report to Congress, 1989," *Morbidity and Mortality Weekly Report* 38, no. 43 (3 November 1989): 743.

Committee on Trauma Research, National Research Council, Institute of Medicine. *Injury in America: A Continuing Public Health Problem.* Washington, DC: National Academy Press, 1985.

Committee to Review the Status and Progress of the Injury Control Program at the Centers for Disease Control. *Injury Control.* Washington, DC: National Academy Press, 1988.

Department of Health and Human Services. *Healthy People 2000: National Health Promotion and Disease Prevention Objectives for the Nation.* Washington, DC: U.S. Government Printing Office, 1991.

Feuerstein, Phyllis. "Incentives Inspire Safe Behavior," *Safety and Health* 145, no. 1 (January 1992): 42–45.

Gordon, J. E. "Epidemiology of Accidents." *American Journal of Public Health* 39, no. 4 (1948): 504–15.

McAfee, R. Bruce, and Ashley R. Winn. "The Use of Incentives/Feedback to Enhance Workplace Safety: A Critique of the Literature," *Journal of Safety Research* 20, no. 1 (Spring 1989): 7–19.

McGowan, Donald E. "The Healthy Way to Reduce Accidents," *Safety and Health* 145, no. 3 (March 1992): 46–50.

Morris, John A., et al. "Mortality in Trauma Patients: the Interaction between Host Factors and Severity," *The Journal of Trauma* 30, no. 12 (December 1990): 1476–79.

Murray, David. "Climb Aboard the 'Healthy People 2000' Bandwagon," *Safety and Health* 147, no. 3 (March 1993): 58–62.

Simpson, Charles W. "The Personal Touch Pays Off in Safety," *Safety and Health* 146, no. 1 (July 1992): 66–69.

Viano, David C. "A Blueprint for Injury Control in the United States." *Public Health Reports* 105, no. 4 (July–August 1990): 329–33.

Vilardo, Frank J. "The Role of the Epidemiological Model in Injury Control," *Journal of Safety Research* 19, no. 1 (Spring 1988): 1–4.

Wolf, Harvey J., and R. John C. Pearson. "Happy Workers Mean Fewer Injuries," *Safety and Health* 145, no. 6 (June 1992): 34–38.

Endnotes

1. Department of Health and Human Services, "Ten Top Leading Causes of Death, 1992," data provided by the National Center for Health Statistics, CDC, *Chronic Disease Notes and Reports* 6, no. 2 (Fall 1993): 1.
2. Department of Health and Human Services, *Health United States, 1991,* DHHS Pub. No. (PHS) 92–1232 (1991): 161–62.
3. National Safety Council, *Accident Facts, 1993 Edition* (Itasca, IL: National Safety Council, 1993), 1.
4. Centers for Disease Control, "Cost of Injury—United States: A Report to Congress, 1989," *Morbidity and Mortality Weekly Report* 38, no. 43 (3 November 1989), 743.
5. National Safety Council, *Accident Facts 1993,* 4.
6. National Committee for Injury Prevention and Control and Education Development Center Inc., *Injury Prevention Meeting the*

Challenge: A Summary (Newton, MA: Education Development Center, 1989), 2.
7. National Safety Council, *Accident Facts 1993,* 111.
8. "1987 Conference on Injury in America: A Summary," *Public Health Reports* 102, no. 6 (November–December 1987), 577–676.
9. Vernon N. Houk and others, "One Fine Solution to the Injury Problem," *Public Health Reports* 102, no. 6 (November–December 1987): 576.
10. National Committee for Injury Prevention and Control, *Injury Prevention Meeting the Challenge,* 2.
11. Lynette Shaw and Herbert S. Sichel, *Accident Proneness* (New York: Pergamon, 1971). For an informative discussion of those studies and papers challenging the concept of accident proneness, read pages 166–216.
12. R. Bruce McAfee and Ashley R. Winn, "The Use of Incentives/Feedback to Enhance Workplace Safety: A Critique of the Literature," *Journal of Safety Research* 20, no. 1 (Spring 1989): 8.
13. Ibid., 9.
14. Ibid., 15.
15. J. E. Gordon, "The Epidemiology of Accidents," *American Journal of Public Health* 39, no. 4 (1948): 504–15.
16. Department of Health and Human Services. *Healthy People 2000: National Health Promotion and Disease Prevention Objectives,* (1991).
17. Ibid., 271–93.

CHAPTER 2

The Home—Injury Occurs in the Privacy of Where We Live

Chapter Outline

Introduction
At-Risk Age Groups
   Children
   The Elderly
Falls—A Major Injury Threat
Selected Danger Areas
   Kitchen
   Bathroom
   Television Set
   Fireplace
Specialized Power Tools and Equipment
   Home Workshops
   Chain Saws
   Lawnmowers
   Snow Throwers
Electricity
Flammable Liquids
Mobile Homes
Holiday Seasons
Summary
Discussion Questions
Suggested Readings
Endnotes

Introduction

As we sit at home watching television, reading a newspaper or magazine, or doing any number of other tasks, the possibility of unintentional injury seems remote. Nearly everyone views the home—be it a house in the suburbs, an apartment on a busy city street, or a room in a house on the edge of campus—as a place of relative safety from trauma. Yet many unintentional injury events, minor and major, occur in and around the home.

    Nearly 20,000 fatalities occur annually in the home resulting from unintentional injury events.[1] A majority involve children of preschool age and senior citizens. For these two population groups, the home is the focus of daily activities: that is, a significant portion of their time is spent each day in the home environment. The most common causes of home-related fatalities are falls, fires, suffocation from ingested objects, and poisoning.

Incidents in and around the home environment cause injuries of differing degrees of severity. Approximately 6 million injuries necessitating emergency medical care occur annually in home-related unintentional injury events.[2] About 80,000 of these injuries result in permanent impairment. These figures cannot be considered totally inclusive because many injuries occur each day that are never reported. If we consider the many small injuries that have happened to us—falls, minor bruises, and cuts that were attended to out of the medicine cabinet first aid kit—it is safe to assume that total injury episodes would amount to many millions more.

The economic consequences of home-related unintentional injury events are extremely high—an estimated more than $85 billion annually. This includes wages lost, medical expenses, property losses from fire, and insurance costs.

At-Risk Age Groups

Although home-related injuries occur to all population groups regardless of age, race, or gender, the vast majority occur to young children and to senior citizens.

Children

The period of time that begins when a child starts to crawl and ends with that youngster's entry into school is filled with possibilities for many different kinds of unintentional injury events. Unintentional injury is the most frequent cause of death for children between infancy and kindergarten—more fatalities than from all other causes of death combined. More than half of these fatalities are the result of home-related circumstances.

Once a child is old enough to crawl, potential hazards materialize. A child must learn what is acceptable behavior and what is dangerous. The infant has no idea of the potential danger of putting a finger into the electrical outlet on the wall. Yet it certainly is fun to explore! Neither is the infant aware of the damage that results from putting a hand on a hot oven window. The bottle filled with kerosene looks like drinking water to the young child wanting a drink.

An awareness of how to live safely at home must be part of every child's learning and growing experience. This process usually results in some pain and tears, but a constant goal must be to see that no serious, long-lasting scars or impairment occurs. Parents and other responsible adults need to take positive steps to help small children through this very important stage of life. This means continual attention to the safety and well-being of the child.

Children learn about safe practices by observing those around them, especially their parents. The parents who habitually fasten their car seat belts before riding out into traffic are going to have a positive effect on a youngster. Families that practice safe daily habits, such as keeping objects off staircases, are setting examples worthy of being followed.

Many safety learning experiences of small children also are of the trial-and-error variety. The child who places a hand on the hot stove is not likely to repeat this action, particularly if the experience is painful. These types of experiences are necessary for young children to transfer learning to other, similar circumstances.

It is important not to underestimate the value of teaching the child explicitly about safety rules and regulations. For example, children must be taught not to run into a street without looking in both directions to assure there is no traffic approaching. Children must be taught not to play with matches. They must learn that there are no exceptions to such basic regulations. Explanation of the rules followed by disciplinary actions when measures are not followed instill safety awareness among preschool children.

Finally, parents and other responsible adults have a major task in identifying and anticipating the numerous potential dangers around the home. One should learn to expect the unexpected when there are young children present. However, the potential hazards in and around the home are not just of concern for preschool children. All ages must be cognizant of the potential for injury-causing situations throughout the home.

The Elderly

Unintentional injury events in the home are common among the elderly. More than 40 percent of home-related fatalities occur to individuals over the age of sixty-five.[3] Although fatalities and long-term injuries among this age group stem from many different causes, the majority result from falls.

Two out of every three fatalities from falls happen to people above the age of 75. There are many reasons for this. Elderly people are less agile and mobile than are younger individuals. As people grow older, sensory perception declines. Loss of sensation in the feet, ankles, and knees may lead to stumbling and difficulty in walking. Reduced coordination contributes to problems associated with balance.

As people grow older, certain physiological changes in bone structure also take place. Bones become easier to break because of a loss of calcium. A fall that for a younger individual might result in a bruise or a minor injury can very easily result in a serious fracture for the senior citizen. Because fractures do not heal as easily in older people as they do in younger individuals, a person of advanced years who suffers a fracture may be incapacitated for a long period of time. Especially dangerous and frustrating to the senior citizen is a broken hip, pelvis, or dominant arm.

Hip fracture is of particular concern for the elderly. Half of the elderly who experience a hip fracture cannot walk normally after the injury.[4] A reported one in eight hip fractures among the elderly results in death from related complications.[5]

The risk of death from falls in general increases with age, especially with people over the age of 85. There are several contributing factors to this increased risk: poor vision, the presence of chronic ailments, and unsteady gait.

In addition to falls, the elderly are at risk for other types of injuries associated with circumstances in the home. Fires present a particularly dangerous situation.[6] The second leading cause of fatality in the home for the elderly is fire and burns. Especially at risk are those over 75 years of age who are invalids or whose mobility is impaired. When trapped in a burning home, such individuals often are unable to escape. As a result, death often occurs from asphyxiation.

Falls—a Major Injury Threat

Although numerous incidents in the home result in fatality and injury to people, falls are the most prevalent. They are the leading cause of nonfatal injury (resulting in over a million injuries each year in the United States) and the second leading cause of injury-related fatalities in the country. Fatalities and injuries from falls impact people of all age groups. While people may be injured in falls at work, school, or in public settings, the majority of deaths and injuries resulting from falls occur in the home.

The concern about injury and death from falls is noted in the federal government health objectives for the nation.[7] This initiative proposes a goal of reducing fatalities from falls and fall-related injuries by the year 2000. In order to achieve this objective, special program emphasis will need to be directed during the 1990s toward at least three population groups at greatest risk: the elderly (ages 65 to 84), the frail elderly (people over 85 years of age), and African-American males between the ages of 30 and 69.[8] A specific objective was also established for reducing the incidences of hip fracture among senior citizens over age 65, so as to reduce hospitalization for this condition.[9]

Understanding the physiological factors that lead to falls offers clues to how such incidents can be prevented. In normal movement, an individual's balance is maintained around the body's center of mass, known as the *center of gravity*. One's center of gravity shifts and changes during various activities and when assuming different postures. However, when a loss of balance fundamentally disrupts a person's center of gravity, a fall results. Such loss of balance can stem from numerous circumstances. For example, an individual might trip over an object in his or her path and fall. The most common kind of fall—a slip—results when someone loses equilibrium and control on a slippery surface, such as an icy sidewalk or a newly waxed floor. Wet surfaces in general present conditions that can cause sudden shift in the center of gravity and lead to a fall.

Many of the safety countermeasures to reduce injury and fatalities from falls have been directed toward environmental factors. For example, those at risk for falls are often encouraged to wear well fitting shoes, rather than floppy slippers or only stockings. To minimize dangers posed by bathroom floors and bath tubs, nonskid bath rugs or mats are encouraged.

Good lighting throughout the home, particularly on stairways and other areas of possible danger, is another important countermeasure to prevent falls. Another safety measure is the removal of objects on the floor that can cause a fall, such as loose rugs, electrical cords, and toys. Basic construction design, particularly of stairways, can serve as an important deterrent as well.

Since most epidemiological studies record the effects of falls but provide lesser information about the causes, more research has been recommended examining the etiology of falls—that is, learning why and how falls cause injury.[10] For example, there is a recognition that prescription drug use is a risk factor that contributes to falls and that use of tranquilizers, sleeping pills, and other antidepressants may double the risk. Still, a great deal more needs to be learned about physiological factors that result in balance abnormality and falls.

Ordinances designed to help reduce the possibility of injury and death resulting from home falls have been legislated. New York City has a law requiring that apartments where young children live must have window guards. Such pioneer legislation can serve as a model to other urban areas where many children live in high-rise apartments and where there is the danger of children falling from windows, ledges, and balconies. Among other things, care must be taken to provide firm window screens and protected outside walkways on the upper stories.

Selected Danger Areas

Within the context of this chapter it would be impossible to provide extensive study of all locations, appliances, and substances that contribute to unintentional injury in the home. Based on overall risk, two rooms—kitchen and bath, appliances common to those rooms, television sets, and fireplaces are singled out for special consideration.

Kitchen

A kitchen can be one of the busiest areas in the home. Even in a small college apartment many activities take place in the kitchen. The various types of electrical appliances found on the counters of nearly every kitchen all have the potential for causing injury. The electric mixer and the blender are examples. Serious injury may result if one's fingers come into contact with the rotating beaters or the cutting blades that are whirling about at high rates of speed.

Gas or electric ranges have potential for serious injury. Of major concern is the possibility of fire. In the case of an electrical range, a burner coil may be left on accidentally and cause serious burns if a person unknowingly comes into contact with the stove. Placing a hand on the hot coil, touching the oven window, or having a skirt or shirt sleeve come into contact with the burner may cause very painful burn injuries.

Gas stoves present similar problems in that any contact with the flame from the burner or the pilot light can lead to a damaging fire. Vapors from flammable liquids, as when gasoline or kerosene makes contact with the pilot light, may lead to an explosion that can destroy the room in seconds, cause an extensive house fire, or cause serious bodily injury.

Another common potential source of fire is spilled grease in an oven or on the stove. Never attempt to extinguish a grease fire by putting water on the blaze. Pouring water on a grease fire will trigger a splashing action that causes the blaze to spread. The flames must be smothered by denying the fire the needed oxygen. A dry chemical fire extinguisher is of greatest value in countering grease fires. Or in the absence of such an extinguisher, if a grease fire begins in a frying pan, turn off the burner and cover the pan tightly with a lid. This will smother the blaze. Pouring baking soda on the flames sometimes has been recommended as a measure to extinguish a grease fire, but extreme care must be taken not to splash the grease when pouring or throwing the baking soda onto the fire.

Most kitchens also contain a variety of smaller cooking appliances, such as toasters, electric frying pans, waffle irons, coffee pots, and corn poppers. Fire may result from the improper use of any one of these appliances, or because of defective heating elements, appliance overheating, or short circuits. Care also must be taken to protect against electrical shock in the operation of any of these electrical devices.

In the case of any cooking appliance, the consumer must use the device in the proper manner. Care should be taken to protect against tripping over electrical cords. Any kitchen appliance or utensil can cause serious problems for small children. Parents can never be too careful in supervising the kitchen activities of their children.

Bathroom

One of the most dangerous rooms in the house is the bathroom. The bath tub and shower stall account for most of the injuries that occur in this room. Because of the combination of soapy water and smooth surfaces of the shower, tub, and floor, falls are very common. Some protection against a fall is afforded by rough-surfaced adhesive strips or suction-cup rubber mats, both of which help to make footing more secure. However, care must be taken since some suction-cup rubber mats may lose adhesion with time and become ineffective. Grab bars mounted on the wall also provide protection against falls.

Extra care should be taken any time a young child is in the bathroom. Particularly among the very young, drownings and scalding can easily occur.

Electrical appliances such as hair dryers and radios often present safety hazards. Electrocutions result from contact with an electrical appliance while one either is in the water or standing on a damp floor. All electrical appliances should be kept away from the bathing area in a bathroom. They should be disconnected when not in use.

Hair dryers are responsible for more than half of all bathroom-related fatalities.[11] It is not uncommon for this electrical appliance to fall into the occupied bathtub and cause an instant fatality. Hair dryers should never be used in a bathtub or while standing with bare feet on a wet floor. It is wise to always unplug the hair dryer when it is not in use. As of 1991, a Consumer Product Safety Commission standard requires that hand-held hair dryers must be manufactured so as not to leak current when immersed in water with the switch in either the "on" or the "off" position.[12]

Television Set

The television set is a standard appliance in nearly every home in America today, with as many as three or four sets per household. Most people give little thought to their possible dangers. Although television has been indicted for many of the social ills in society today, it is rarely seen as having potential for direct physical harm. At least two concerns should be highlighted in this respect, radiation and fire.

There has been much debate over the potential effects on humans of radiation given off by color television sets. X-ray emissions that are in excess of the standard limit established by the federal government may be released. This emission, which passes through the front of the color picture tube, occurs under conditions of failure of certain receiver components. The television set will usually continue to function normally and the amount of radiation emitted is of a low level. Nonetheless, concern and differences of opinion exist as to the effect of exposure to such low-level radiation over extended periods of time. There is always potential danger from any new amount of radiation in the environment, and every effort should be made to avoid introducing any new radiation hazards.

The second major concern with television usage is fire. An estimated 10,000 fires a year, some resulting in injury and death, occur from television sets. Very high voltages of electricity run through a television set and any contact may result in electrical shock. Also, placing the television set near a radiator may result in a buildup of heat within the cabinet and start a fire.

Many home fires traced to television sets are the result of electrical malfunctioning. It has been reported that some fires have been caused by the "instant-on" feature. This problem can be avoided by purchasing instant-on sets with a switch that can cut the current. In addition to issues of electrical malfunctioning, more fires occur with sets encased in plastic cabinets.

Because a television set fire is electrical in nature, it is important that the electrical current be disconnected. Water-based fire extinguishers should not be used in trying to put out such a blaze. Instead, it is best to use a dry chemical fire extinguisher.

Associated with a television set in many homes is an outside antenna located on or alongside the house to improve reception. Many electrocutions have resulted from contact with these antennas and nearby electrical power lines. Extra care must be taken in putting up or repairing an antenna. If the antenna comes in contact with overhead power lines, the potential for electrocution is present.

Fireplace

Many hours of enjoyment are experienced sitting, reading, playing, and talking around the fireplace. However, measures must be taken to protect against starting a potentially disastrous blaze. The National Fire Protection Association estimates that each year some 14,000 home fires begin from fireplaces.

House fires often begin from sparks thrown off by the fire in the fireplace. Certain woods that are burned, particularly freshly cut wood, are more likely to propel sparks potentially hazardous distances. Every fireplace should have a spark screen to cover the opening completely and provide protection from a possible house fire.

Care also must be taken when igniting the blaze in a fireplace. Never should any kind of flammable liquids be used to start or rekindle a fireplace fire. Even an apparently dying fire may explode into a dangerous inferno if a container of flammable liquid, such as gasoline or lighter fluid, is left open near the fireplace.

The chief cause of fireplace-related house fires is an overheated or defective flue—the passage in the chimney through which air to the fire and smoke from the fire pass. A flue should be constructed with a flue lining. Failure to use such a lining often results in disintegration of the mortar and bricks, creating a potential fire hazard. An undersized flue may cause a smoky fireplace and also poses a potential danger. The flue and the chimney should be cleaned and examined regularly.

Before seasonal use begins or at any sign of problems, the structural components of the fireplace should be checked by a qualified inspector. Damaged mortar or broken bricks must be repaired before any fire is started.

A properly constructed fireplace must have a damper. Normally, a damper is made of cast iron and has a hinged lid that can be opened and closed to regulate the draft. It can also prevent loss of room heat when there is no fire in the fireplace, an especially important factor in cold weather. Keeping the damper closed in summer can help prevent insects from entering the house through the chimney. The damper should not be closed until one is positive that any fire is totally extinguished. Otherwise poisonous carbon monoxide may accumulate in the room.

It is unwise to burn trash and paper in a room fireplace, as the embers are likely to settle on the roof after leaving the chimney and start a fire. Embers also may become trapped in the upper part of the chimney and cause a blaze within the chimney structure.

Many people use artificial logs, usually made from sawdust and wax, in the fireplace. Since these artificial logs can produce a tremendous amount of heat, only one should be burned at a time. Care must be taken not to come into personal contact with the burning wax of the artificial log, as this may result in serious injury and burns.

Children should never be permitted to poke around a fire with fireplace tools. Care must also be taken not to wear clothing that might be easily ignited when one comes into proximity of the fire in the grate.

Specialized Power Tools and Equipment

In most households one can find a variety of power tools and equipment. Some are purchased to help reduce the amount of labor necessary to carry out various tasks around the house and yard, such as cutting the grass, trimming the bushes, and shoveling snow from the sidewalk. Other equipment is for recreational and creative activities of interest to the occupants, such as woodworking equipment like saws, grinders, and drills. Every type of power tool and equipment, whether electrical or gas operated, has the potential for causing unintentional injury and fatality. It would be impossible to present a discussion of the safety features of every type of power tool and equipment found around our homes. Therefore, several have been singled out because of special safety concerns or popularity of use.

Home Workshops

Many people dream of having a workshop in their home where they can go after a long, hard day at work and relax. Most often the workshop is located in the garage or in the basement of the home. Unfortunately, unintentional injuries related to the use of equipment in a home workshop are common. Of particular concern are those pieces of equipment that are power operated. Power saws, drills, grinders, and soldering guns are examples of equipment that can cause serious injuries.

Two basic types of injuries are normally noted in such home workshop settings: wounds resulting from contact with the cutting surface of the power tool and electrical shock injuries. Anytime that a cutting power tool is used, a blade guard must be on the machine and be in use. After shutting off the power, do not move a hand toward the blade or cutting surface until the tool has come completely to a halt. Injuries can also be reduced by using a saw blade that is sharp and cuts clean.

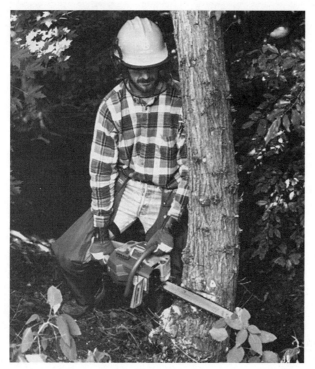

When held properly the chain saw is a safe power tool for use in the woods.

In the presence of children, all power equipment should be shut off when an adult is not present. Children should not be permitted to activate the equipment when there is not proper supervision.

Any electrical power tool should not be used without the three-pronged plug. To help protect against electrical shock, the operator of power equipment should make sure that the cord is insulated properly and not frayed.

When workshop equipment is located in the basement or the garage, the possibility of dampness around the working area arises. An individual should not stand in a damp area when operating power tools.

Chain Saws

Chain saws are used around homes for cutting trees and for clearing shrubs and other brush. The chain rotates, at a very high rate of speed, and it is contact with this chain mechanism that causes serious injuries.

It is estimated that as many as 36,000 persons a year need treatment in an emergency room for chain saw injuries. The number of such

> **WORK NOT APPROPRIATE FOR CHAIN SAWS**
>
> 1. Do not have another person hold the wood as it is cut.
> 2. Do not cut small flexible branches.
> 3. Do not cut closely spaced branches.
> 4. Do not cut with a chain saw from a ladder.
> 5. Do not climb a tree to cut a branch with a chain saw.
>
> ---
>
> Source: U.S. Consumer Product Safety Commission, *Consumer Information Guide: Chain Saws* (Washington, DC: U.S. Government Printing Office, n.d.).

injuries seems to have decreased since the early 1980s.[13] This is due to implementation of a Consumer Product Safety Commission regulation issued in 1985 designed to reduce the incidence of chain saw kickbacks that often result in injury. A chain saw kickback can occur when the tip of the blade touches any object or when the wood being cut closes in and pinches the saw in the cut.

The regulation now requires that all saws must have a guard to shield the hand closest to the blade and a chain brake which stops the blade in a fraction of a second if the saw should kick back. Tip guards on the end of the guide bar that protect the nose of the chain saw from kickback are also required.

It is important that the chain saw operator uses proper operating procedures. The saw should be started on a firm surface. It should be carried with the chain pointing away from the body and operated with both hands on the saw at all times. It is very easy for the saw to jump and cut a finger or hand if it is not being held firmly. If the saw jams or binds in the wood, it may kick backward toward the operator. Such a situation may result in very serious bodily injury, particularly to the face. Contact with the muffler should be avoided, as very serious burns can result from touching the heated muffler.

The person using a chain saw must dress appropriately and safely. Gloves should be worn to protect the fingers and hands. Heavy, sturdy shoes are useful in providing protection for the feet. Safety glasses or goggles protect against flying debris. One should never wear loose-fitting clothing that could get caught in the rotating chain.

Chain saw injuries occur to the experienced user as well as to the novice. Regardless of the degree of one's experience with this tool, care should always be taken to prevent a serious and painful injury.

Lawnmowers

Today most homeowners have a motorized lawnmower. Some are pushed by hand, others are riding mowers; some are run electrically, most are run by gasoline. In each instance there is potential for injury.

It is estimated by the Consumer Product Safety Commission that by the early 1990s, about 19,000 individuals were treated annually for injuries from power lawnmowers. This is a reduction from close to 50,000 such injuries in the early 1980s. A major reason for this improvement in number of injuries associated with operation of lawnmowers is due to a government regulation in 1982 mandating that all lawnmowers be equipped with a device that stops the blade when the operator releases the handle.

Injuries resulting from lawnmower operation commonly occur as the result of contact with the rotating blade, from contact with flying objects propelled by the blades of the machine, and from the overturned riding mower used on uneven terrain.

Most people use rotary blade mowers. These kinds of lawnmowers are much more efficient than are the reel-type mowers. However, they also are much more dangerous, in part because of the rotating blades, which reach speeds of 200 miles per hour. In the absence of a safety guard over the chute, objects can be hurled as projectiles some distance.

Push mowers must have a rear guard which helps to prevent feet and hands from coming into contact with the rotating blade. Another safety feature is a guard which directs the discharge opening downward. This helps to reduce the likelihood of objects being hurled from the opening.

Much of the protection from injury-producing circumstances related to lawnmower operation is the responsibility of the operator. One should never remove any of the safety features that are now required before a manufacturer can sell a machine.

Certain rules apply to safe operation of the lawnmower. The operator of a lawnmower should dress appropriately, avoiding loose clothing which could become entangled in the rotating blade. It is also important to prepare the area where mowing is to occur. Any objects that the mower could throw as a projectile and injure someone should be removed before beginning the mowing.

The operator must disconnect the spark plug wire any time the mower is held upright to check the blade. This also is important when cleaning grass from the blades area because turning the blade by hand may start the engine.

When refueling the mower, it is important to assure that the muffler and engine have had time to cool. Explosive fire can result if these parts of the machine are still hot and gasoline is spilled on them.

Riding mowers present several unique concerns. Before mounting or dismounting a riding mower, make sure that the blades are shut off completely. There is no law which regulates blade stop time for riding mowers. The blades usually rotate for an average of three to four seconds after the power has been shut off. Most mowers today have a switch in the seat that shuts off the engine when the blades are engaged and the operator leaves the seat.

Riders should never be permitted to accompany the riding mower operator. This is particularly true of small children. A second rider can easily fall from the machine and be injured.

When mowing on an unlevel surface with a riding mower, mow up and down the slope. If using a push-type mower, mow horizontally across the slope. Do not use a power mower on steep slopes and take particular care not to mow on wet grass. It is easy to slip on such surfaces.

There is an increase in the use of electric mowers. Special care must be taken not to cut or run over the electrical wire, so when using an electric mower, mow away from the electrical outlet. Also, one should never cut wet grass using this type of mower as a short in the electrical cord could result in electrocution.

Snow Throwers

The use of snow throwers, useful labor-saving devices for removing snow from driveways and sidewalks, has become increasingly popular. Since their introduction in the latter part of the 1960s, these have become widely used machines. The machine has a fast moving auger which bites into the snow bank and tosses the snow a distance, out of the way.

This machine can be very dangerous when operated without proper care. The Consumer Product Safety Commission estimates that there are over 3,000 snow thrower related injuries annually.

Snow throwers have a number of safety features designed to protect the operator. The most dangerous component for the operator is the chute from which the snow is blown. Any chute large enough to blow snow is large enough to accommodate a hand. Injury is usually the result of a person attempting to dislodge impacted snow from the discharge chute. Operator carelessness is the primary risk factor resulting in hand injuries.[14]

Most manufacturers of snow throwers now produce them with deadman controls. This is a mechanism which shuts off the auger and drive when the handle is released. As a result, the possibility of coming into contact with the operating blade is lessened.

CASE PROJECT—ESTIMATING WATTAGE DANGERS

To apply these concepts, consider the household use of an electric frying pan that requires 1,200 watts. Normal household voltage is 120 volts. Using the formula (watts = volts × amperes) the amount of electric current flowing through the pan is ten amperes. Because less than one ampere of current can be fatal, any electrical appliance is a potential danger.

Electricity

Most people fail to understand the basic concepts of electricity. They do not realize that flowing through the electrical system of their homes is enough electrical current to cause a destructive fire or death from electrical shock. It is important that we not only understand how electricity works but that we learn to respect its use in the home. While there has been a decrease in electrocutions in industry in recent years, there has been an increase in such incidents around the home. This is due in part to the increased use of electrical appliances and power tools in our society.

It is the current or electricity flowing through an electrical wire that can kill a person or create enough heat energy to start a fire. The flow of current is measured in *amperes*. The current flowing through a wire is moved along by a force known as a *volt*. Extremely high voltage is generated at an electrical power plant. By the time the current has reached a home electrical circuit, it has been transformed to approximately 120 volts. The rate at which an appliance uses electrical power is measured in *watts*. A watt is the rate of using amperes pushed along by a certain number of volts. Most electrical appliances list their watts usage. Household light bulbs, for example, generally range from 25 to 300 watts.

The normal wall outlet is capable of carrying fifteen amperes. If the current exceeds fifteen amperes, the circuit is overloaded. When this occurs, the house wiring becomes overheated and an electrical fire may ensue.

The human body is an excellent conductor of electrical current. When an electrical circuit is *grounded* adequately, the current passes through the body and goes into the earth or ground. Passage of current through one's body may produce fatal shock or serious burns along the pathway traversed by the current or may result in cardiac arrest. Electricity will take the path of least resistance. In the human body this is most likely to be the blood vessels and the nerves.

For this reason, it is important to use appliances adapted so that the body cannot become a grounding pathway. Any electrical appliance or electrical power tool should either have double insulation construction or a three-pronged grounded plug. These features protect against electrical current that can leak into the outer shell of the appliance or power tool. Otherwise when a person's hand touches the appliance or tool, that individual becomes part of the pathway for the electrical current.

Current may be carried directly to the ground by the third prong on a plug—which means any leaking electricity runs through the grounded third wire. The third prong on an appliance should always be used. Never cut it off or use the appliance when the prong is broken, as removal eliminates the grounding safety feature for the electrical current.

Electrical wall outlets should be designed to accept three-pronged plugs. If they are not, use a two-pronged adapter. Attach the "pigtail" third wire to the screw holding the faceplate to the wall receptacle. If this third wire is not grounded, the electrical current will have no grounding place except through the body of the individual in contact with the appliance. An individual should consider installing a three-pronged outlet when an adapter is not available.

Many homes are now built with ground fault circuit interrupters (GFCI). GFCIs detect any leakage of electrical current in a circuit. They are designed to shut off the electricity when a leak is detected. Power can be restored by pressing a reset button when the electrical leak has been eliminated.

Ground fault circuit interrupters are installed in place of standard outlets. Often their installation is found near sinks or other places where there is water. When an electrical appliance such as a hair dryer or an electrical tooth brush is dropped in the water, the GFCI will immediately shut off the electricity, thus preventing electrocution.

Where there is a GFCI it should be tested regularly, at least once a month, to assure that it is working properly. In homes not having this device, it should be a priority that at least one portable plug-in GFCI be purchased for the bathroom sink area. They are inexpensive to purchase—usually less than twenty dollars.

Electricity's properties make it highly dangerous to the human heart. Electrical shock may cause a condition known as *ventricular fibrillation* when a current crosses the heart. In this condition the heart fails to pump blood normally. Heart function may be so affected that there is no blood movement to or from the heart.

There are two different kinds of electrical current, alternating current (AC) and direct current (DC). Alternating current is capable of producing ventricular fibrillation at very low voltage. When a person comes into direct contact with AC they may not be able to let go. With direct current the individual can usually let go of the appliance or source of the electricity.

Even a very small amount of electrical current, such as that which comes from a house electrical wall outlet, may lead to ventricular fibrillation. Bare feet or standing on a wet surface greatly magnifies the possibility of this happening.

When such electrocution occurs, careful measures need to be taken. The rescuer rendering emergency aid to the victim must not personally become exposed to the "locking-on effect" that often occurs. This situation occurs when a person attempting to rescue a victim who is in contact with the electrical current becomes "locked on" by the same current and is unable to let go. As a result, the person rendering emergency care also becomes a victim of electrocution.

Never touch an individual who is in contact with an electrical wire until the current has been shut off or until the circuit has been broken. If these measures cannot be taken, then the victim must be removed from the source of the electrical current with utmost caution, using strong, dry wooden sticks or boards or heavy cardboard. One should never touch the victim while wet or in contact with other conductors of electrical current, such as aluminum or other metals.

Once victims are separated from the electrical current, they are likely to require cardiopulmonary resuscitation (CPR). This will be the case if there is no evidence of heartbeat or breathing. The purpose of CPR is to continue the flow of blood through the circulatory system while the heart is not functioning normally. If the blood is not circulating throughout the body and carrying oxygen to the various vital organs, particularly the brain, death occurs. When used properly, CPR may stimulate a return of normal heart rhythm. Cardiopulmonary resuscitation involves exerting pressure that squeezes the heart between the sternum and the vertebrae. Many lives have been saved through proper use of CPR. However, serious complications can occur when CPR is applied improperly. For this reason, it is important that every person should be trained in the proper application of CPR by appropriately certified CPR instructors.

In addition to circulatory problems, burns over any part of the body can result from direct exposure to electrical current. Usually the

> **CASE PROJECT—HOME ELECTRICAL CURRENT CONTROL**
>
> Every person should know how to shut off the current in a place of residence. This demands knowledge of which fuses on the master fuse box control the electrical current to the various rooms, appliances, and other parts of the house. Examine the fuse box of the house or apartment where you live. Learn what procedures you would need to take to shut off the current flowing throughout your particular place of residence.

first sign of burns is a gray or yellow discoloration. Because it is impossible to ascertain the depth of the burn, a victim of severe electrical shock must see a physician as soon as possible.

Not only is it important to know various precautionary measures to protect oneself and others from electrocution, but it is also helpful to know how one can best survive for several hours, or even several days, *without* electricity. Ice storms, blizzards, and strong winds often cause downed power lines and electrical outages. In these circumstances one very quickly learns how dependent our society is on electrical power.

Lack of electrical service can range from that of simple inconvenience—as when people are without lights for a short period of time or when a computer screen goes blank resulting from a short, quick electrical outage—to more serious occurrences. The latter results when individuals living in all-electric homes find themselves without heat in extremely cold temperatures for lengthy periods of time or without water when private wells operated by electrical pumps cease to function.

Spoilage of food in refrigerators and freezers can occur when there is an absence of electricity for a period of time. During these emergencies, refrigerators and freezers should not be opened more than is absolutely necessary. Without electrical power, a closed freezer will keep food frozen for two to three days. For longer periods of time, dry ice may be needed to keep the food from spoiling.

Flammable Liquids

Located in and around nearly every home are numerous liquid flammable substances that can be extremely dangerous. Many of these liquids can be ignited from a spark or flame at some distance from the

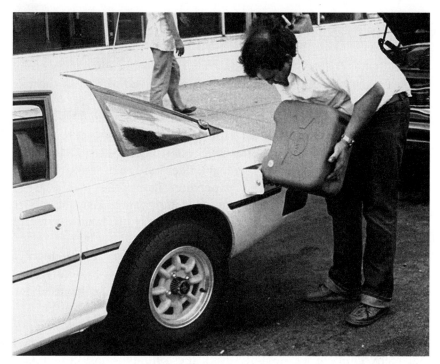

Gasoline is often kept in garages and sheds in gasoline containers. It is important that gasoline, which is highly flammable, be stored in a shed away from the house. Also gasoline should only be stored in approved containers.

container. Such liquids give off vapors that are heavier than air—hence, the vapors are capable of flowing along the floor. When they come into contact with some flame or spark, such as the pilot light on a furnace or hot water heater or a discarded cigarette, explosion may result.

One of the most commonly found flammable liquids in the garage or shed area is gasoline. Most people have a can of gasoline available for use in the lawnmower, the chain saw, the snow thrower, or other gasoline-powered machines. Yet we often give little thought to the fact that this exposure to gasoline may be every bit as lethal as having a stick of dynamite or some other explosive in the home. Gasoline is highly flammable and can ignite with explosive force that may result in serious injury, fire, property loss, and death.

If it is necessary to store gasoline in a container, make sure that the can is designed specifically to store gasoline safely, with the contents properly labeled. This means that there should be a pressure-release valve as well as a flame arrester. It is particularly dangerous to store gasoline in glass jars or other breakable containers. One should never leave the gasoline can open. Not only may the fumes be ignited, but there is danger of an individual, particularly children, ingesting the liquid.

It also is a dangerous practice to carry gasoline containers in the trunk of a motor vehicle. Should a car be involved in a crash there is the possibility of an explosion. The potential for fume leaks from the trunk into the car presents another very serious condition. One is traveling in a "tinder box" ripe for explosion.

Another dangerous practice that often occurs around charcoal grills involves the pouring of charcoal lighter fluid on the burning coals. If people pour lighter fluid on such open fires, flames can quickly spread from the grill to their hands and arms. It is important to keep the lighter fluid can away from burning coals in a charcoal grill, bonfires, or any open flames.

Lighter fluid or electric starter coils should be used only initially to start the charcoal burning. Once the fire is started, it is very dangerous to add more fluid. At no time should gasoline be used for lighting charcoal grill fires.

Not only must concern be expressed regarding the explosive potential of gasoline and other flammable liquids, but it must be noted that many children accidentally drink these fluids—most commonly, young children. They see the fuel in a cup or can and mistake it for water and begin to drink. Ingestion of flammable liquids may cause the individual to gag, a sign that something is wrong. If any of the fluid gets into the lungs of the individual, serious illness or death may ensue. For example, as little as one teaspoonful of kerosene may cause death.

The importance of proper storage of all flammable liquids cannot be overemphasized. All must be kept in a cabinet or storage shed away from enclosed living quarters of the home. There must be adequate ventilation to permit any vapors to escape safely into the atmosphere. Properly constructed cans should be the only place that such liquids are kept. It goes without saying that such liquids be stored out of the reach of children.

Mobile Homes

Several million people in the United States live in mobile homes. For many young couples, the mobile home presents a comfortable, affordable place to live until they have enough money to purchase a permanent home. Mobile homes also are very popular among retired senior citizens, particularly in states such as Florida and Arizona. Upkeep and maintenance is minimal and there is adequate living space for two people.

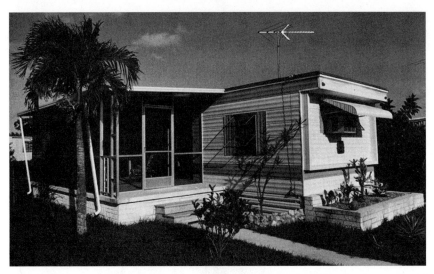

Mobile homes provide a comfortable place for many people to live. Measures should be taken to protect against fire since many injuries and fatalities occur to individuals caught in mobile home fires.

Though the mobile home is a very comfortable place of residence, it does present a number of dangers. It is particularly vulnerable to high winds, heavy rainstorms, and fire. In the case of a tornado or hurricane, mobile trailers may be blown off their foundation blocks and found some distance from where they were standing. There is danger in any heavy windstorm of trees being uprooted and blown onto the mobile home, which has little structural protection against such circumstances. As protection against windstorms, a mobile home should be tied down after placing it on the foundation blocks.

Many people reside in mobile homes located in the same generalized area. These neighborhoods are often referred to as mobile home parks. Every mobile home park should have some type of early warning system, so that when high winds are anticipated, mobile home occupants can take proper precautions. Prearranged safety measures should include the presence of an alternative place of shelter. For example, permanent structures that have basements and reinforced roofs should be identified where the occupants can go for protection. If there is no prearranged location where individuals can go during a tornado warning, occupants should leave their trailers and lie down in a depression or ditch in the surrounding terrain at the approach of the tornado.

Fire has a tendency to spread very rapidly through a mobile home. This is due in part to the basic design of a mobile home—narrow corridors and low ceilings. Some of the materials used in trailer home construction, such as plywood paneling, are highly flammable.

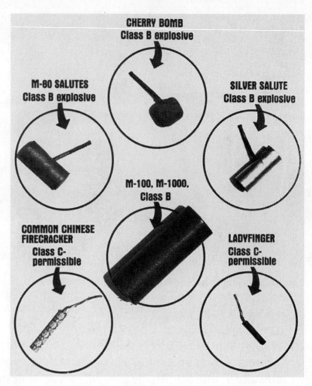

Fatalities occur as the result of using fireworks. The CPSC has banned a number of fireworks that have caused blindness, finger or hand amputation, injury, and death. Examples of such illegal fireworks are shown here. In contrast, the common Chinese firecracker and ladyfinger contain less than 50 milligrams of powder and are legal in most states.

The basic construction design of a mobile home often prohibits easy escape. Windows in particular are not useful as emergency exits. Normally, trailer windows are smaller and many are jalousied, with shutter-like obstacles that impede escape. Some window installations should be able to serve as escape routes, particularly those in mobile home bedrooms. Every mobile home should be equipped with smoke detectors and should be occupied only if the facility has at least two unobstructed doors.

Holiday Seasons

Unintentional injury events can occur any day of the year and at any time during the day or night. However, certain holiday celebrations present an increased potential for injury.

> **RULES FOR FIREWORK SAFETY**
>
> 1. Never let children play with fireworks.
> 2. Read and follow all instructions on the label.
> 3. Light fireworks outdoors away from houses and flammable materials.
> 4. Keep a bucket of water nearby when using fireworks.
> 5. Do not try to relight or handle malfunctioning fireworks.
> 6. Never ignite fireworks in a glass or metal container.
> 7. When lighting fireworks, keep people out of range of possible injury.
>
> Source: Committee on Injury Prevention and Control, Academy of Pediatrics, "Children and Fireworks," *Pediatrics* 88:652–653, 1991.

The Fourth of July has long been celebrated with fireworks displays. Fireworks can cause severe burns, injury to the eyes, hands, and fingers, loss of limb, and fatalities. The Consumer Product Safety Commission reports more than 12,000 fireworks-related injuries requiring emergency hospital treatment occur each year. Two-thirds of these occur during the month of July, centering around the holiday.[15]

Among preschool children sparklers are the leading cause of injury. Firecrackers, sparklers, bottle rockets, and twisters cause injury among individuals of elementary and junior high school age. Among older teens and young adults injury is most likely to occur from firecrackers and bottle rockets.[16] Although both boys and girls are injured, the most injuries occur to young males.

Many types of fireworks—including cherry bombs, aerial bombs, and large firecrackers—have been banned in some localities. Local, regional, and state laws and ordinances banning fireworks have been passed. However, the laws and their enforcement tend to be inconsistent from one locality to another. There have been initiatives to ban fireworks of every type at the national level. However, such national bans have not been successful, due to objections raised by the fireworks industry and other pressure groups. A total ban of fireworks would probably lead to increased illegal sales. Today, government regulations permit the use of fireworks in general community displays. However, those organizing such displays must adhere to local fire and safety regulations. Generally commercial fireworks displays do not result in injury to people.

Halloween is another holiday season in which many unintentional injuries occur. Children must not be permitted to wear Halloween costumes which are flammable. They should also wear costumes which are

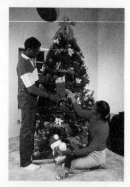

All too often the happiness of the Christmas holiday season is ruined by a tree fire. Every family should take care in the selection and decoration of their tree to prevent a disastrous or destructive fire.

easily visible to motorists, since injury often occurs when drivers do not see the children as they cross the streets during their trick-or-treat activity. All children must be taught to use sidewalks, not the streets, when out making their rounds.

Halloween masks that are worn by children can cause suffocation or impede vision. Parents should be careful that the masks do not affect breathing or obstruct vision, and that they can easily and quickly be removed.

At Halloween time homeowners often place candles in jack-o-lanterns. These should be kept well away from contact with clothing and other costume fabrics worn by children. Children should never carry jack-o-lanterns that are illuminated with candles.

Unfortunately, there are reports every Halloween season of children being given tainted or poisonous treats. Measures must be taken to alert the youngsters of these potential dangers. It is a wise measure that children be required to bring the treats home before they are permitted to eat any of them. Parents or other responsible adults can examine the treats to assure they have not been tampered with in any way.

In many communities police departments and other public safety agencies offer to x-ray treats for the purpose of detecting any foreign objects. There is increasing development of alternative activities for children by community agencies to serve as another option to trick-or-treating at Halloween.

The Christmas season is another time of joy, family gathering, fun, and goodwill for many people. It is, however, a time of increased likelihood of injury-producing situations.

Nearly every home and many business establishments display a decorated tree at this time of the year. Many of these are natural trees, capable of igniting very easily. It is important when purchasing a live tree that it be freshly cut. The drier the tree, the more serious the potential for fire. Many trees that are purchased a week or two prior to Christmas were actually harvested up to two months previously. These trees are usually dry enough to be a serious fire hazard even before they are purchased.

As a protective measure one should never buy a tree that is shedding needles. Tapping the tree on the ground will indicate if the tree is too dry for safe use in the home. Fresh needles will not break when bent between the fingers. Once needles begin to fall off, that tree should be removed from the home, as it is dangerously dry and could burn rapidly with the slightest exposure to a spark or flame. There is no reliable method of flameproofing natural trees.

Increasing numbers of people are purchasing artificial trees made of plastic or metal. The likelihood of fires with these trees is reduced.

However, care must be taken not to place electric lights on the metal portions of these trees. When lights are attached with a frayed cord, the entire tree may become electrically charged.

All lights used at the Christmas holiday season should be inspected for safe operation. Light sets should include the Underwriter Laboratory (UL) mark to indicate that the manufacturer constructed the light set according to industry safety standards. All lights, indoor and outdoor, should be checked for frayed wires and broken sockets. Any lighting set that is damaged should never be used.

One should never use combustible decorations, such as candles, around a tree. Another hazard is the use of spun glass, "angel hair," and artificial snow. These trimmings are nonflammable when used individually. However, if artificial snow is sprayed on angel hair, it may burn very rapidly when ignited.

Summary

Even though it normally is a place of comfort and enjoyment, the home is not always a safe place to be. Many circumstances that result in injury and even death occur in and around the home. No room or section in the home is free from the possibility of injury. The kitchen and the bathroom are two rooms in which injury-producing situations are most likely to occur. Also, one can find a variety of tools, equipment, and appliances, such as lawnmowers, power tools, and snow removal equipment, which have the potential for causing various degrees of injury.

Unintentional injuries at home occur most commonly among two population groups: young children and senior citizens. For both population groups the home is where they spend a majority of each day. Among the elderly, falls are a major cause of injury. Because of the inquisitive nature of preschool children, there are numerous daily situations that present the possibility of injury.

Around a home there are numerous possibilities for situations that can result in electrocution. Measures must be taken not only to protect against electrocution, but to know what to do to assist another person who has sustained an electrical injury.

Holiday seasons have great potential for injury. The Fourth of July is a time when many individuals are injured from various explosives, firecrackers, and other fireworks. Halloween is a time when children dress up in costume and go about their neighborhoods, leading to further injury risks. At the Christmas holiday season the possibility of fire is increased with the presence of trees, lights, and other decorations. At all holiday seasons measures need to be taken to protect against injury and property destruction.

Discussion Questions

1. Why do the majority of home injuries and fatalities occur among children and the elderly?
2. What physiological changes occur as an individual grows older that result in increased risk of injury?
3. Discuss the health objectives for the nation by the year 2000 relating to falls.
4. What are several countermeasures that can be used to help reduce injury resulting from falls occurring in the home?
5. What are several potentially dangerous objects that one can find in the kitchen?
6. What types of dangers relate to the television set?
7. Identify and discuss various power tools and what measures can be taken to protect against injury from their use.
8. Explain the principles involved in electricity.
9. What is the difference between alternating and direct current?
10. What is the ground fault circuit interrupter (GFCI)?
11. Where electrocution has occurred, what precautionary measures should an individual rendering emergency care take?
12. Give examples of flammable liquids. In what ways are they dangerous?
13. Discuss various measures that can be taken to improve the safety of individuals living in mobile homes.
14. What are several potentially dangerous products associated with the Fourth of July celebration that can cause injury?
15. Identify measures that should be taken to protect against injury, fatality, and fire during the Christmas and Halloween holiday seasons.

Suggested Readings

Barnwell, Mary, and Warren Galke. "An Epidemiologic Analysis of Fatal Home Accidents in North Carolina," *Journal of Environmental Health* 49, no. 4 (January–February 1987): 208–13.

Centers for Disease Control. "Fatal Injuries to Children—United States, 1986," *Morbidity and Mortality Weekly Report* 39, no. 26 (6 July 1990): 442–51.

"Chain Saws: Now They're Less Fierce." *Consumer Reports* 55, no. 5 (May 1990): 304–09.

"Combustion Appliances and Home Safety." *Consumers' Research* 75, no. 5 (May 1992): 30–34.

Committee on Injury Prevention and Control, American Academy of Pediatrics. "Children and Fireworks," *Pediatrics* 88, no. 3 (September 1991): 652–53.

Consumer Product Safety Commission. "No. 35: Portable Hair Dryers," *Product Safety Fact Sheet* (1990).

Duda, Marty. "Closing the Gait on Slips, Trips, and Falls," *Safety and Health* 141, no. 6 (June 1990): 48–51.

Ertas, A., and others. "Design and Development of a Fall Arresting System," *Journal of Safety Research* 21, no. 3 (Fall 1990): 97–102.

Fisher, Leslie. "Childhood Injuries—Causes, Preventive Theories and Case Studies," *Journal of Environmental Health* 50, no. 6 (May–June 1988): 355–60.

Miller, Barrett C. "Falls: A Cast of Thousands Cost of Millions," *Safety and Health* 137, no. 2 (February 1988): 22–26.

Miller, Timothy P., and Reid H. Hansen. "Snowblower Injuries to the Hand," *The Journal of Trauma* 29, no. 2 (February 1989): 229–33.

Pearlman, Cindy. "How to Avoid Household Falls," *Safety and Health* 149, no. 2 (February 1994): 76–78.

Planek, Thomas W. "Home Accidents: A Continuing Social Problem," *Accident Analysis and Prevention* 14, no. 2 (February 1982): 107–20.

Pollock, Daniel A., Daniel L. McGee, and Juan G. Rodriguez. "Deaths Due to Injury in the Home among Persons under 15 Years of Age, 1970–1984," *Morbidity and Mortality Weekly Report* 37, no. SS-1 (February 1988): 13–20.

Seward, Paul N. "Electrical Injuries: Trauma With a Difference," *Emergency Medicine* 24, no. 8 (15 June 1992): 157–68.

"The Hazards of Faulty Home Wiring." *Consumers' Research* 75, no. 6 (June 1992): 32–35.

Tideiksaar, Rein. "Falls Among the Elderly: A Community Prevention Program," *American Journal of Public Health* 82, no. 6 (June 1992): 892–93.

Endnotes

1. National Safety Council, *Accident Facts, 1993 Edition* (Itasca, IL: National Safety Council, 1993), 98.
2. Ibid.
3. National Safety Council, *Accident Facts 1993,* 100.

4. Barrett C. Miller, "Falls: A Cast of Thousands Cost of Millions," *Safety and Health* 137, no. 2 (February 1988): 22–26.
5. Ibid.
6. A discussion of fires is found in chapter 4.
7. Public Health Service, *Healthy People 2000: National Health Promotion and Disease Prevention Objectives* (Washington, DC: U.S. Government Printing Office, 1991): 276.
8. Ibid.
9. Ibid., 279.
10. A. Ertas and others, "Design and Development of a Fall Arresting System," *Journal of Safety Research* 21, no. 3 (Fall 1990): 97–102.
11. Consumer Product Safety Commission, "No. 35: Portable Hair Dryers," *Product Safety Fact Sheet* (1990).
12. Ibid.
13. "Chain Saws: Now They're Less Fierce," *Consumers Report* 55, no. 5 (May 1990): 304–09.
14. Timothy P. Miller and Reid H. Hansen, "Snowblower Injuries to the Hand," *The Journal of Trauma* 29, no. 2 (February 1989): 233.
15. Committee on Injury Prevention and Control, American Academy of Pediatrics, "Children and Fireworks," *Pediatrics* 88 (1991): 652–53.
16. Ibid.

CHAPTER 3

Consumer Safety—Careful Purchasing of Items for Household Use

Chapter Outline

The Consumer
The Consumer Product Safety Commission
   The Legislation
   Commission Activities
National Electronic Injury Surveillance System (NEISS)
Working Relationships between CPSC and Other Agencies
Consumer Product Concerns
   Flammable Fabrics Act
   Fabric Flammability
   Consumer Product Labeling

Aerosols
Poisoning
   Causes of Poisoning
   Poison Prevention Packaging Act
   Impact of Regulation
   Aspirin Poisoning
   Poison Prevention Measures
   Poison Control Centers
Toy Safety
Summary
Discussion Questions
Suggested Readings
Endnotes

The Consumer

Everyone regardless of age, gender, or race is a consumer. Rarely does a week pass without an individual purchasing some product for the home, college dormitory room, or apartment. The choice might be an item of clothing, some appliance for use in the kitchen, a tool for use in the workroom or the garage, or a toy for a child. These and innumerable other purchases make major contributions to the American economy.

However, many of these purchased items bring with them the potential for causing injury, disability, and even death. Many common products we have in our garages or the places where we live may be serious safety hazards. Over 33 million persons are injured annually in situations associated with consumer products. Within this total, some 29,000 fatalities occur and 110,000 persons are permanently disabled. The estimated costs of such injuries are approximately ten billion dollars.[1]

In some instances the product itself may be hazardous. It may be toxic, as are many of the household cleansers and flammable liquids kept in the closet or the garage. Other products might not be thought of as hazardous, yet certain parts can cause serious injury. This is the case with many children's toys, such as a baby's rattle. No one would deny an infant a rattle, yet the small pebbles that create the rattling sound can lead to a choking death if the rattle breaks and the pebbles lodge in the throat of the youngster.

Increasing concern over the lack of protection available to the consumer in the United States has led to the formation of a number of consumer advocate and protection groups. Some of this interest has centered around protection against unfair economic factors. Price gouging, lack of product quality, and other unfair "rip-offs" of customers have resulted in increased awareness of the rights of the consumer. The matter of consumer rights also includes the importance of guaranteed merchandise—including guarantees of freedom from unwarranted danger. Products should be useful and work properly for whatever the intended purpose. Moreover, no consumer should be personally endangered unnecessarily by the purchase and use of a product.

Consumer safety is a matter for which the consumer, as well as the manufacturer, must accept responsibility. The consumer has a right to be assured that the manufacturer will not produce a dangerous item. On the other hand, many defects may not be discovered until the products have been purchased, brought home, and used. The consumer must be alert to potential product defects. Feeling a frayed wire, noting a chip in the glass, or smelling the odor of smoke from the motor of an electric appliance may alert one to a product defect. Assurance of consumer safety cannot be relegated to someone else. Both the manufacturer and consumer have specific roles in providing a safe consumer environment.

Along with the manufacturer and consumer who work together to assure the safety of products, the federal government has become involved in consumer safety endeavors. Federal government, in the form of the Consumer Product Safety Commission, establishes regulations, sets guidelines, and recommends standards for a variety of consumer products.

The Consumer Product Safety Commission

In 1972 the United States Congress passed legislation known as the Consumer Product Safety Act. This legislation was designed to provide the consumer with a reasonable amount of assurance that a product, when purchased, is safe and reliable.

The Legislation

The basic mandate of this federal law has been to protect the consumer from unreasonable risk of injury from consumer products. Provisions of this act created a regulatory agency—the Consumer Product Safety Commission—which reports directly to Congress. This federal government commission has jurisdiction over more than 15,000 consumer products.

The Consumer Product Safety Act also was designed to encourage the establishment of safety standards for the manufacture of a number of consumer products. It was anticipated that the establishment of various standards would reduce the risk of consumer injuries and fatalities stemming from normal product usage.

The definition of a consumer product regulated by this legislation has been rather broad. Any article manufactured for use in or around the home or school, for recreational purposes, or in other similar situations is considered a product of concern to the Consumer Product Safety Commission. Examples include bicycles, children's toys, furniture, appliances, power tools, and lawnmowers. Several products identified specifically in the legislation that were not to be the responsibility of the commission included firearms, alcohol, tobacco, food, drugs, cosmetics, motor vehicles, airplanes, boats, and poisons such as insecticides, fungicides, and rodenticides. Other agencies of the federal government have responsibility for regulation of these products.

Commission Activities

The Consumer Product Safety Commission is authorized to carry out several different functions. The commission issues and then enforces mandatory product safety regulations, designed to ban unsafe products from the marketplace. Products may be removed from commercial sale that do not comply with mandated standards. The commission also has authority to initiate product recall programs. Public information initiatives are another important activity of the commission.

Setting Product Standards

It is the responsibility of the Consumer Product Safety Commission to investigate and analyze potential hazards to ascertain whether a safety danger exists. Because it is impossible to investigate every consumer product sold in American commerce, each year priorities are established for the commission as it investigates products and establishes standards. Usually priority will be placed on products which have been associated with deaths and injuries.

Based on the collection and analysis of data, hazardous products are identified. Data are collected from a variety of sources as the commission carries out its investigations. One source is the National Electronic Injury Surveillance System (NEISS) which collects information from hospital emergency rooms throughout the nation. Also data are obtained from death certificates and accident investigations carried out by the regional offices of the Consumer Product Safety Commission. Another source of information comes from consumer complaints. This process leads to an identification of those products for which it is felt that mandatory safety standards need to be established.

The public must be informed of any plans to establish a mandatory standard. All public groups—citizen and consumer groups, as well as individuals—have the opportunity to provide input into the standard setting process.

Upon establishing and issuing of a standard, it then is the responsibility of the commission to monitor consumer product sales and to assure compliance.

Seizure and Removal

The commission has authority to seize and remove from the marketplace products that are in noncompliance with published standards. Criminal prosecution can be initiated against companies manufacturing such products and against individuals selling them. Because of the threat of prosecution, many products are voluntarily recalled by the manufacturing company. It is estimated that more than 2,300 voluntary recalls involving more than 168 million products have taken place since the original passage of the legislation.[2]

Product Recall

The Consumer Product Safety Commission uses enforced product recall quite extensively. The purpose of such recalls is to remove potentially dangerous products mandatorily from the marketplace. Recall activities involve products that are directly dangerous as well as those which display poor workmanship in their manufacture.

Public Information

A number of different measures by the Consumer Product Safety Commission alert consumers of potentially dangerous products. The commission uses public information initiatives, including the mass media and other public information networks, to reach the general public. Educational efforts both inform the public of the benefits of purchasing certain products, as in the case of home smoke detectors, or of the possible danger of certain consumer-bought products. Labeling on a number of consumer products has been used to warn the public of potential dangers of incorrect or improper use.

Industrial Cooperation

The Consumer Product Safety Commission also works with industry to encourage voluntary redesign and manufacture of consumer products. In close relationship with business and industry, the commission encourages the establishment of voluntary product safety standards. Recognizing the importance of manufacturing products that are not inherently dangerous to the users, many companies have voluntarily worked to improve the safety quality of their products.

Administering Other Federal Laws

In addition to the duties established as a result of the 1972 consumer legislation, the Consumer Product Safety Commission has been given the responsibility of administering various regulations and standards set forth in four other federal laws:

1. The Flammable Fabrics Act
2. The Federal Hazardous Substances Act
3. The Poison Prevention Packaging Act
4. The Refrigerator Safety Act

National Electronic Injury Surveillance System (NEISS)

A major mission of the Consumer Product Safety Commission is to investigate the causes of product-related fatalities and injuries, and then to develop recommendations for prevention. The collection and analysis of data needed to accomplish these tasks is the primary role of the National Electronic Injury Surveillance System (NEISS).

NEISS is a computerized clearinghouse that provides information about product-related injuries on a daily basis. This data collection is accomplished by the monitoring of 64 sample hospital emergency rooms located throughout the nation. Data compiled from these selected hospital emergency rooms are used to estimate national incidences of injuries and fatalities. Members of the Consumer Product Safety Commission review the data, and from this information, specific problems of concern are noted for which further study and investigation are necessary.

Information from data collected by the NEISS system is available for review and analysis by the general public. A publication entitled *NEISS News* disseminates this information.

Working Relationships between CPSC and Other Agencies

The Consumer Product Safety Commission has not been without its critics and detractors. Because of its various legislative mandates, this federal regulatory agency has reached directly into the home and life of almost every American. For this reason, none of us can be indifferent to the presence and workings of this agency. We must question how effective its activities have been in decreasing the numbers and incidences of consumer product-related fatalities and injuries.

It is important also that this powerful regulatory agency not work in isolation from other agencies and organizations involved in matters related to consumer safety. The Consumer Product Safety Commission needs to cooperate with existing state and local programs designed to improve product safety. Many states and local agencies conduct similar activities in research, establishment of standards, and education of the public. It should not be a goal of the CPSC to replace these programs and activities with a federal bureaucracy.

CPSC initiatives must also be carried out in cooperation with the private sector, particularly the business and industrial communities. Too often business and industry view governmental regulatory agencies as nothing more than "policing" organizations of the federal government. Somehow, through cooperative measures, activities must be designed to bring together the private sector and the CPSC to create a safer environment for all consumers.

Consumer Product Concerns

Each day we are exposed to consumer products that have potential for causing death and injury. Possibly the most common exposures are to fabrics such as clothing and the upholstery of furniture. Not only must we become informed about measures that protect us from injury from various products, we also need to be aware of the warning labels required to inform the public of possible dangers.

Flammable Fabrics Act

Enacted originally in 1953, the Flammable Fabrics Act was designed to ban the manufacture and sale of highly flammable fabrics used in the manufacture of clothing. This legislation authorized the Department of Commerce to set various manufacturing standards and gave this agency of government the power to enforce those standards.

Several years later this legislation was amended to cover a wider range of wearing apparel such as gloves, hats, and footwear. A number of interior home furnishings such as carpets, rugs, mattresses, and mattress pads were also included.

Fabric Flammability

Clothing fires often cause severe burn injuries. Fire victims generally suffer more serious burns on those parts of the body that are covered with clothing than on uncovered areas. In short, the extent of injuries resulting from burning of flammable fabrics is a serious problem.

Several factors are considered in determining the flammability of a particular fabric. Clothing burns at different rates, because textiles used in the manufacture of clothing have different burning characteristics. These differences should be known. The kind of fiber, the weight and weave of the fabric, the surface of the fabric, and the design of the garment all determine flammability.

When considering the degree of flammability of a particular fabric, two factors are particularly important: the ease of ignition of the material and the rate it will burn. For the most part, these two properties are inversely proportional to the weight of the fabric. In other words, the lighter the fabric, the more easily and rapidly it will burn; heavier fabrics are not as likely to burn. For example, wool garments are comparatively fire resistant. They ignite, but then usually burn slowly, and often extinguish themselves when the source of ignition has been removed. But although such heavier fabrics do not burn as easily or as rapidly as do lighter garments, when ignited they do generate more heat.

Synthetic fibers such as nylon and polyester are usually less flammable than are lightweight cotton materials. Such synthetics burn slowly and often self-extinguish when removed from the source of the fire. A particular problem with many synthetic fibers is that they tend to melt when hot, and the melted, liquid fibers cause serious burns.

Many clothes are a combination of synthetic and natural fibers. These garments will burn at the same rate and with the same intensity as the natural fiber. For this reason, a polyester-cotton blend fabric will probably be as flammable as an all-cotton shirt.

Close-fitting garments are not as likely to burn as are loose-fitting ones. Loosely woven clothing permits greater exposure to oxygen and greater danger of fire. Larger air spaces help to support combustion. Pajamas, robes, flared skirts, and blouses with ruffles and large sleeves are very flammable. A fluffy, deep-pile garment will burn faster than will a closely knit, low-pile one.

The weave of the fabric will also cause variance in the flammability of a garment. The tighter the weave, the less likely it is to burn.

Flame-Retardant Clothing

Federal regulations require that children's sleepwear be flame retardant. All children's pajamas, nightgowns, robes, and other sleepwear must meet standards prepared by the Consumer Product Safety Commission. Not only must the sleepwear be flame retardant, but it also must be so labeled.

Specific laundering procedures are required for washing flame-retardant fabrics. For example, flame-retardant finishes of cotton fabrics will be lost if they are laundered improperly. Warm water (between 105 and 120 degrees Fahrenheit) is the best temperature for washing flame-retardant clothing. Excessively hot water often causes the fabric to wrinkle; low heat also should be used in drying these fabrics.

Soap and bleach may damage a garment's flame-retardant qualities. Chlorine bleach renders the flame retardant totally ineffective. Soap leaves a fat deposit buildup on the fabric that affects the retardant negatively. The same is true of the use of certain fabric softeners.

Labels that give proper laundering instructions now appear on sleepwear for children. Warnings about certain products and washing procedures are also included. Because of the complexity of these instructions and the lack of consumer education, many people ignore the recommendations.

It must be understood that flame-resistant fabrics are not flameproof. They will burn when in contact with a flame. However, they should burn slowly and self-extinguish when the source of the fire is removed. Burns will still occur if the clothing is not removed or if the fire is not extinguished immediately.

In spite of the importance of using flame-resistant fabrics in the manufacture of clothing, there has been concern about certain products putting the user at risk for serious other health problems. For example, during the 1980s the Consumer Product Safety Commission banned the sale of TRIS-treated sleepwear. TRIS is a flame-retardant chemical which was widely used in the manufacture of children's sleepwear. Research evidence linked this chemical to higher cancer incidence—that is, TRIS may be carcinogenic when an individual experiences long-term exposure.

Furniture Upholstery

Fires involving upholstered sofas and furniture result in several thousand deaths and injuries annually. Measures have been taken in the past several years to improve the nonflammability of these household items.

Particular concern has centered around developing products that are resistant to fire ignition by cigarettes. Many injury-causing fires are started when an individual falls asleep in a chair or on the sofa while smoking, or when a discarded cigarette falls on these types of furniture. Consumers should make certain when purchasing upholstered sofas and chairs that labeling on the furniture indicates fire resistant materials have been used.

Consumer Product Labeling

The Consumer Product Safety Commission has authority under provisions of the Federal Hazardous Substances Act to require that warning labels be placed on many consumer products. The purpose of labeling is to warn consumers about hazards of a particular product. Following identification of potential dangers of a given item, warning labels indicating the hazard must be made available. In addition, pertinent safety information must be present on the box or container in which the product is sold.

Labeling of products includes the use of such words as "danger," "warning," or "caution." Toxic substances are to be labeled "poison" and have the skull and crossbones symbol on the container.

Instructions for rendering first aid care and for the safe handling and storage of the hazardous substance must appear on the labels.

Another purpose of labeling is to inform consumers how to install a product safely. When an item must be assembled by the consumer, there are measures that must be taken to ensure that the product operates in a safe manner.

Instructions may need to be present on the product to indicate how much can be used safely. A typical case is the use of certain types of household cleansers. Acid-type drain cleaners serve useful purposes; however, too much of this cleaner can damage the pipes, and the acid content eventually will destroy them.

Products that are considered to be hazardous and covered by provisions of the Federal Hazardous Substances Act fall into six different categories:

1. *Toxic products* are agents which can produce personal injury or illness when ingested, inhaled, or are absorbed through the skin.
2. *Corrosive substances* include anything that can cause destruction of living tissue upon direct contact. This destructive action occurs through chemical action on the skin.
3. *Irritants* are any noncorrosive substances that produce local inflammation of the skin upon prolonged or repeated contact.
4. *Strong sensitizers* include any substance to which a person becomes allergic after exposure. Upon initial exposure usually no ill effects are noted. However, subsequent exposures result in strong allergic reactions.
5. *Flammability points* are points at which substances will burn, referred to as the combustion or flammable level.
6. *Pressure* is the generation of force when a substance is exposed to heat or subject to decomposition. This pressure buildup may cause injury or illness.

Aerosols

A number of consumer products found around the home come in pressurized cans. It is estimated that over 2 billion aerosol cans are sold in the United States annually. Serious injury can be caused if these cans are stored or discarded improperly. An aerosol can that is thrown into a fire may explode; a can stored in a hot environment—such as near a stove or oven or in the sun—may explode at a temperature of 120 degrees Fahrenheit. Obviously one should never leave such cans in a car parked in the sun when the temperature inside the vehicle may become very high on a hot, sunny summer day.

Care should be taken when discarding aerosol cans. Even if the can appears to be empty, there may be enough pressure to cause an explosion. For this reason, the can should not be disposed of with any burnable trash.

Some of the contents found in aerosol cans may be toxic. Aerosol sprays may result in dizziness, nausea, skin irritation, headache, blurred vision, and other physiological problems. People have died as the result of exposure to aerosol propellants. Respiratory problems, cancer, and heart trouble have been associated with these sprays.

Anyone using aerosol sprays should pay attention to the warnings on the can. One should also make sure that there is ventilation in an indoor room because of the toxicity of these spray propellants.

Poisoning

Numerous agents are found around the home that are poisonous to humans. Approximately 6,000 fatalities occur each year as the result of ingesting poisonous substances.[3] In addition, several hundred thousand individuals are treated in hospital emergency rooms each year for accidental ingestion of poisonous substances and products.

Though poisoning is a condition that affects all age groups, it is of particular concern among children. Mortality associated with poisoning among children has decreased during the past decade; however, morbidity is still extremely high. As many as 700,000 cases of poisoning are reported annually to the poison control centers.[4] Recognition of this has led to identifying the reduction of nonfatal poisoning emergency room treatments as a national health and safety objective to be achieved by the year 2000.[5] Children four years of age and younger have been singled out in this objective as particularly at risk.

Causes of Poisoning

Poisoning can occur as the result of exposure to a variety of different substances. Some common causes are household cleaning agents, medications, foods, and liquid poisons.

Household Cleaning Agents

In most homes there are numerous cleaning agents, such as toilet bowl cleansers, furniture polishes, kitchen drain cleansers, and other types of soaps and cleansers. When ingested orally, most of these can cause serious injuries.

All cleaning agents used in a home should be kept out of reach of children, not only when stored but when they are in use as well. It is not uncommon for a cleansing agent to be left unattended with the safety cap removed. Little imagination is needed to understand the potential danger if a child spots the uncapped bottle.

Many individuals are unaware of the potential danger of common household cleansers. For example, a highly corrosive drain cleaner is a potentially dangerous product found in most households. Extensive damage can result when a highly corrosive drain cleaning agent is swallowed or splashed into the eyes. It might be wise to purchase a granular drain cleaner rather than a liquid. At least if the cleanser is spilled accidentally, the granular type may be brushed from the skin before damage results. The liquid type is more difficult to remove; if the skin is wet, tissue destruction normally begins immediately.

Household users of chemicals must consider wearing rubber or plastic gloves for protection. When such a substance is spilled on the skin or splashed in the eyes, immediately wash out the eyes with running water for 10 to 15 minutes. If the corrosive drain cleaner is ingested, do not attempt to make the victim vomit. In all such cases, contact a physician or hospital emergency room immediately.

It is necessary that individuals be aware of the potential dangers associated with mixing two or more cleansers together. Ammonia, which is found in many household cleaning products, can cause irritation of the eyes, nose, and the skin. When mixed with bleach, however, a highly irritating gas is released. One should never mix chlorine bleach with ammonia or toilet bowl cleansers. If such a mixing does occur, the individual should immediately leave the room and go to where there is a fresh oxygen supply (outdoors is best).

All household cleansers must, by law, carry instructions about the proper emergency procedures to take in case of a spill. Note these directions before using the cleanser and follow them completely.

Medications

Medications, both prescription and over-the-counter, are a major type of home poisoning. Much has been said and written about the importance of keeping medicines out of reach of small children. Though there is much concern about children getting into medicine cabinets and ingesting medicines, more than half of all fatalities from medication poisoning occurs to adults. This is because older people tend not to read labels on their medications, fail to follow proper instructions, and establish patterns of taking medicine out of habit without checking whether they are reaching for the appropriate bottle. In spite of this, proper storage of all medications must be maintained, so that children cannot get to them. It is also important that all medicines be properly labeled so that no one, either child or adult, takes an inappropriate amount of any medication.

Foods

A number of foods are, in and of themselves, poisonous to humans, such as certain types of mushrooms and shellfish. Food poisoning also results when certain foods have been inappropriately refrigerated and as a result have become spoiled. Bacterial action on some foods results in salmonella, a very common type of food poisoning. It is nearly impossible to obtain accurate data indicating the amount of food poisoning that occurs in the United States; however, it is reported that each year there are several deaths.[6]

Food must never be stored on the same shelf or in the same cabinet with cleaning products. The potential for taking a can of some poisonous substance instead of soup or other food item is great enough to prohibit such practices.

Liquid Poisons

There are many liquid agents that are poisonous. Of particular note are various petroleum distillates which, when swallowed, can cause internal damage to the various organs of the body. Serious burns can also result when such substances come in contact with the skin. Other poisonous liquids include lighter fluid, furniture polishes, turpentine, and products containing lyes and acids.

An all too common practice is leaving gasoline containers unattended—especially when people fill the lawnmower and then go out to mow the lawn. The justification for leaving the gas can unattended in the garage or yard? Since more gas will be needed before the mowing is completed, why not have it available? The tragic potential for injury in these situations is obvious, particularly if small children are present.

Poison Prevention Packaging Act

In 1970 the United States Congress passed legislation aimed at protecting people, particularly small children, from poisonous substances found around the house. A number of toxic and dangerous products are now covered by regulations developed under mandate of this legislation. Examples include petroleum distillates, such as cigarette lighter and charcoal lighter fluid, and fluid for use in lanterns. Batteries containing sulfuric acid are also regulated, along with antifreeze, turpentine, and various liquid furniture polishes. In 1991 regulations were issued for household glues, artificial fingernail removers containing acetonitrile, and hair wave neutralizers containing sodium or potassium bromate. Administration of these various regulations is the responsibility of the Consumer Product Safety Commission.

Regulations have been established which require that medications be packaged in such a manner that would prevent young children from opening them. Children of preschool age are particularly susceptible to poisoning because this is a period of time when they learn through exploration. They touch and taste whatever is available. Youngsters at this age are unable to differentiate between candy and multicolored pills and medicines, or between water and a cup of paint thinner. The law requires that medicine and toxic substance containers be designed to make it difficult for the child to open them. These safety caps are not always child-proof. They do slow down access by the child, however.

Some exceptions should be noted. Regulations under provisions of this legislation permit the use of containers without safety packaging for some prescription medications such as antibiotics and nitroglycerin. It permits the sale of some over-the-counter medications without safety packaging. Provision is also made for adults to request that a physician or pharmacist not use safety packaging. Medications may be sold in nonsafety-proof packages only if a warning is carried on the label.

Impact of Regulation

Child-resistant packaging of toxic household substances has had a positive effect in reducing the number of fatalities and injuries from oral poisoning. In spite of the fact that the sale of products in child-resistant containers has been useful in reducing the number of poisonings, there are related problems. With the increased difficulty in opening child-proof containers, many individuals have broken the container or the cap, either purposely or accidentally. Still others, once they have opened the containers, leave them open, increasing the availability of

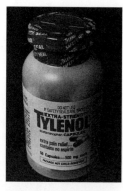

Federal regulations mandate that over-the-counter medications be sold in safe, child-proof containers.

poison to small children. Some people have transferred the contents of the containers to other bottles that either have no labels or inappropriate labels.

Liquid medications tend to gum up and increase the difficulty of opening the cap. Another problem exists with non-English speaking individuals who are unable to read the warning directions or the opening directions on the container.

It has been reported that despite the mandates of this legislation, 43 percent of medications that are found in the household setting are without safety packaging.[7] Obviously, such use of containers without safety packaging circumvents the intent of the law and increases the risk of poisoning to children.

Aspirin Poisoning

Aspirin is probably the most commonly used home drug. It is safe when used according to instructions. Aspirin is especially useful in countering various types of pain including headaches, high fevers, and other types of physical stress. It is very effective in alleviating some of the symptoms associated with arthritic conditions. Most individuals have taken aspirin at some time in their lives.

Because of the common use of this drug in our society and the basic mentality that suggests one should "take an aspirin" for almost any ailment, people often do not realize the potential danger associated with taking too many aspirins. Each year thousands of people overdose on aspirin, resulting in the need for emergency care and in a number of fatalities.

Aspirin was the first product singled out in the early 1970s for safety packaging under provisions of the Poison Prevention Packaging Act. Aspirin poisoning is a particular risk factor for children of preschool age. Children have been taught by their parents that taking aspirin when needed is good for them. In an effort to encourage the child to take the medicine, parents will say such things as "it tastes just like candy." These statements of encouragement to the child only contribute to the problem of aspirin overdose at a time when the child is left unsupervised and the aspirin bottle is within reach of the youngster.

Whenever an individual has ingested an overdose of aspirin, it is important that immediate emergency care be obtained. The signs and symptoms of aspirin overdose often are not present immediately. Many times the best sign or indication of aspirin poisoning is the presence of an empty or partially empty bottle. When this occurs, efforts should be taken to remove the aspirin by encouraging vomiting of the contents of the stomach. Medical attention is particularly important at this time.

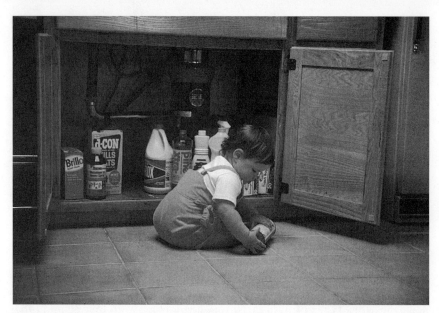

Poisons need to be kept out of reach of all children.

Poison Prevention Measures

There are numerous activities designed to protect against poisoning. Since young children are particularly at risk, the importance of proper and safe storage of all potentially poisonous substances is to be noted. These substances, particularly medications, should be kept in their original containers with childproof caps in place. Children should be taught the dangers of ingesting poisonous substances.

The need to reduce the number of individuals using emergency rooms for treatment of poisoning was noted in the national health objectives initiative for the year 2000.[8] Children under the age of four were specifically targeted by this initiative, since it is estimated that more than 107,000 children of preschool age are treated annually in hospital emergency rooms for poisoning.[9] As a result of the initiative, various community agencies concerned about public poison education and prevention will be implementing programs in the 1990s designed to help achieve the proposed poisoning reduction goals.

The importance of poison prevention initiatives also has been recognized formally by the United States Congress. Congress has authorized the president to designate the third week in March as National Poison Prevention Week (Public Law 87–319). Every year during this week, community agencies, schools, industries, and other interested organizations are encouraged to develop poison prevention programs designed to alert the general public of the dangers associated with ingestion, inhalation, and absorption of poisonous chemicals.

The point is not just to list all, or even a significant number, of the steps one might take to "safety proof" the home, but to educate the general public about household poisons. An awareness of the potentially toxic substances found in everyday use around the home is imperative. Out of awareness comes a desire to take whatever measures are necessary to protect persons from such hazards in the home.

Poison Control Centers

Such a vast array of poisonous substances may be found that it is difficult for any single medical practitioner to be adequately informed about more than a few. As many as a quarter million toxic products are on the consumer market. Some of these include label information about the toxic ingredients in the product. However, this is not the case for all items.

To treat poisoning cases, information regarding a specific toxic substance must be known. To meet this need, a number of poison control centers have been established throughout the United States—the first in Chicago in 1953. At that time, a pilot project was initiated by the Illinois Chapter of the American Academy of Pediatrics in combination with several other interested agencies and some twenty major hospitals.

The center in Chicago and other early poison control centers were established to serve medical personnel, mainly physicians. Although some centers still only provide information to physicians, many serve other individuals seeking information regarding poisoning.

These centers have several purposes: (1) increase public awareness of potentially hazardous substances; (2) provide information regarding the ingredients, toxicity, expected poisoning signs and symptoms, and recommendations for treatment of poisons and medicines; and (3) provide a twenty-four-hour telephone hotline service.

Each center has information for every known poisonous substance. Information is available about the composition of the poison, measures to be taken to neutralize the toxic effect, and other pertinent data. In addition, each poison control center has reference material on poisoning.

In the mid-1980s there were over 300 poison control centers located throughout the United States. By the early 1990s this number had been reduced to less than 100 as the result of increasing focus on regionalization of the centers.[10] Today poison control centers must have round-the-clock staffing and be certified as meeting criteria published by the American Association of Poison Control Centers. A listing of these centers is published annually in the journal, *Emergency Medicine*.[11]

In spite of the attempt to provide coverage to the entire United States population, there are localities which do not have the available services of a poison control center. A recommendation by the Third National Injury Control Conference, sponsored by the Center for Environmental Health and Injury Control of the Centers for Disease Control and Prevention, stated that state and local governments should provide poison information via toll-free telephone service to people who do not have access to poison control centers.[12]

Toy Safety

The sale and manufacture of toys are big business in the United States, with nearly two billion toys being sold annually.[13] A toy is a source of much joy to a child. Most adults also experience warm feelings when they give playthings to a child. During such happy times one seldom thinks of the potential for injury. Yet thousands of children are injured annually from toys.

The Consumer Product Safety Commission estimates that 148,000 individuals annually receive hospital emergency room treatment for injuries associated with toys.[14] Half of these injuries are to children under the age of five. It is important to emphasize that adults must take the responsibility for helping to protect children from injury resulting from dangerous toys.

People do not seem to respond to safety as a selling point when purchasing toys for their children. In purchasing a toy for a child, the age and skill level of the youngster must be considered. Is the toy acceptable and recommended for the age of child to whom it is to be given? Only toys that suit the skill and ability levels of the child should be purchased. Age recommendations are now required to be placed on many different types of children's toys. For example, all electrical toys now have labels indicating the earliest age at which a child can be expected to use the toy safely.

Toys with electrical components create potential for thermal burns and electrical shock. Electric toys must be constructed properly so as to eliminate the possibility of shock. This means that the toy must be wired properly and meet specific requirements for maximum surface temperatures. Any toy with heating elements is not recommended for use by children under eight years of age.

Several other hazards are associated with toys. Toys with sharp edges and points can cause serious cuts, stabs, and wounds. Many seemingly innocent toys such as dolls may have pins or wired interior structures that can be dangerous. Lacerations, contusions, and abrasions are the types of injuries most frequently reported from exposure to toys.[15]

Toys with small movable parts that can be swallowed, inhaled, or placed in the ear or nose by a child are particularly dangerous. Choking is an often noted occurrence resulting from playing with these types of toys. Choking incidences involving balloons and small parts of toys cause a majority of fatalities related to children's toys.

Impaired hearing often results from exposure to the loud, concussion-type blasts of cap guns. Boxes of caps now must be labeled with a warning that they should not be used indoors or within one foot of the ear. In 1989 a manufacturing company, in cooperation with the Consumer Product Safety Commission, removed caps which were shown to ignite prematurely if dropped or by friction when carried in a pocket.

Toys that look like weapons or that can be propelled either purposefully or accidentally have potential for injury causation. Several different types of toys serve as projectiles or have movable parts that may fly through the air. In 1988 the Consumer Product Safety Commission banned the sale of lawn darts as toys. These heavy metal darts are tossed at a ring on the ground. Often used by both adults and children as a recreational activity, the game led to thousands of injuries and several deaths before being banned.

Nonpowder firearms that employ compressed gas to propel darts, steel BBs, and lead pellets are sold as toys to adolescents between the ages of eight and eighteen. Toy guns (of the gas-, air-, and spring-operated variety) are examples. Nearly 2.5 million such weapons are sold each year in the United States; over half are sold to children under 15 years of age. Often these objects are not perceived as dangerous. They are considered by some parents as toys that children should have. However, most of the time they are used with little adult supervision.

The Consumer Product Safety Commission has recommended that children under the age of fourteen not use high velocity BB or pellet guns. So far the commission has not developed any regulatory mandates. Several states have passed laws restricting the sale and use of these firearms. Such regulations include a few that require a permit for possession and usually limit sale to children over eighteen.

Archery equipment, toy bows and arrows, and sling-propelled toys contribute to injuries. A major concern with projectile-type toys is the practice of intentionally aiming the toy at another person. This is particularly true for guns used in play. Toy guns, as well as BB and pellet guns, bows and arrows, and archery equipment, should never be aimed at another person.

> **TOYS RECALLED BECAUSE OF CHOKING POTENTIAL—1990**
>
> 1. Solid-color plastic whistles—whistles break apart and could be ingested by a child.
> 2. Doll and baby bottle sets—bottle caps and nipples present a choking hazard to children.
> 3. Solid-color siren whistles—made of plastic, they are easily broken apart releasing small parts with potential for choking.
> 4. Fun bus—a yellow bus with various parts has a thin band of decorative plastic with letters and numbers. This decorative plastic band has been removed by children and has caused choking.
> 5. Press 'N Roll Boat—plastic multicolored bathtub boat with moveable wheels posed a choking hazard.
>
> Source: *News From CPSC*, various releases, January–March 1990.

Riding toys are associated with more injuries necessitating hospital emergency room care than any other type of toy. Most such injuries result from scooters, tricycles, and wagons.

Once a toy has been purchased, the parent or responsible adult should be aware of the condition of the toy. A broken toy may present potential for serious injury. Also toys with moving parts must be handled properly. Such toys require continuing supervision.

The storage of toys is another concern. Many injuries result from falls which occur because of improper storage. A toy left on a stairway may be all that is needed to trigger a fall. Children should be taught and encouraged to store their toys in a designated location when not in use. This not only protects people from falling over them, but also prevents a broken and damaged toy.

Approximately 70 percent of all toys sold in the United States are imported. The leading manufacturer of toys sold in the United States is China. That fact makes it particularly difficult for the Consumer Product Safety Commission to police toy construction, since a U.S. regulatory commission has no enforcement authority over foreign manufacturers. Therefore, the most effective measure to enforce mandatory regulations is to carry out recalls from the distribution stores where the imported toys are sold.

Summary

Every day thousands of products are purchased for use around the home that have potential for injury-causing circumstances. It is estimated that more than 33 million persons are injured annually from interaction with consumer products, with some 29,000 fatalities resulting.

Recognition of the need for consumer safety protection led to the passage in 1972 of the Consumer Product Safety Act. This legislation created a commission and guidelines for establishing regulations of product safety. Subsequent legislation centered on four areas of concern: the Flammable Fabrics Act, the Hazardous Substances Act, the Poison Prevention Packaging Act, and the Refrigerator Safety Act. The Consumer Product Safety Commission has responsibility to set mandatory standards for a variety of products. It also may issue recalls of products considered to be dangerous. The commission may issue labeling requirements for products to warn of dangers and also carries out a variety of educational initiatives to inform the public of potential dangers to their safety.

To assist the Consumer Product Safety Commission in its many activities, the National Electronic Injury Surveillance System has been established. NEISS is a clearinghouse that provides information about product-related injuries. Data collected by this system are useful in identifying products needing regulatory attention.

The flammability of fabrics is a consumer issue that has received much attention. The fiber, weight, and weave of fabrics impacts the cloth's flammability. Measures have been taken to assure increased safety of fabrics for clothing, furniture, rugs, bedding, and other household objects.

Poisoning cannot be overlooked as a household hazard. Measures have been taken to safety proof our homes from numerous toxic substances. Today many toxic substances are required to be sold in packaging that will make it difficult for children to open. Poison control centers have been established to provide information about the toxic ingredients of all poisonous substances, including measures to take to neutralize the toxic substance.

The sale of toys is big business in the United States. Numerous regulations and recalls have taken place in an attempt to provide a safer environment for children playing with toys.

Discussion Questions

1. Who has the responsibility for safety of consumer products?
2. What has been the basic result of the legislative mandates of the Consumer Product Safety Act?
3. Discuss the various responsibilities carried out by the Consumer Product Safety Commission.
4. What is the process by which the Consumer Product Safety Commission sets consumer product standards?
5. What four federal laws are administered under provisions of the Consumer Product Safety Act?
6. What is the National Electronic Injury Surveillance System (NEISS)?
7. In what ways does the Consumer Product Safety Commission work with other state and local agencies and the private sector for safety of the consumer?
8. What are various factors in determining the flammability of a fabric?
9. Although synthetic fibers burn slowly, they present serious problems related to burns. Why is this?
10. Why is there a need to package prescription drugs in special protective containers?
11. What are the poison control centers?
12. Why is aspirin poisoning such a problem?
13. What are some of the safety factors associated with the sale of aerosols?
14. What are some factors that make children's toys dangerous?
15. A majority of toys sold in the United States are imported. What problems does this create for consumer safety regulation?

Suggested Readings

Christoffel, Tom, and Katherine Christoffel, "Nonpowder Firearm Injuries: Whose Job is it to Protect Children?" *American Journal of Public Health* 77, no. 6 (June 1987): 735–38.

Consumer Product Safety Commission. *Poison Prevention Packaging: A Text for Pharmacists and Physicians.* Washington, DC: U.S. Government Printing Office, n.d.

Dawson, Carol G. "Choosing Safe Toys for Children," *Consumers' Research* 73, no. 12 (December 1990): 15–16, 40.

"Education Efforts Promote Product Safety." *Safety and Health* 145, no. 1 (January 1992): 23–25.

Gulaid, Jame A., and others. "Household Survey of Child-Safe Packaging for Medications," *Public Health Reports* 105, no. 4 (July–August 1990): 430–32.

Planek, Thomas W. "Home Accidents: A Continuing Social Problem," *Accident Analysis and Prevention* 14, no. 2 (February 1982): 107–20.

"Playing for Keeps: Kids, Toys, and Dangers." *Consumer Reports* 55, no. 11 (November 1990): 716–19.

Poison Prevention Week Council. *National Poison Prevention Week: Editor's Fact Sheet, 1994*. Washington, DC: U.S. Government Printing Office, 1993.

"Unintentional Poisoning Mortality—United States, 1980–1986." *Morbidity and Mortality Weekly Report* 38, no. 10 (17 March 1989): 153–57.

Endnotes

1. U.S. Consumer Product Safety Commission, *Who Are We, What We Do,* no. 103 (Washington, DC: U.S. Consumer Product Safety Commission, October 1988): 1. Unless otherwise noted, data used in this chapter are from various Consumer Product Safety Commission public releases dated between 1990–1993.
2. Ibid., 6.
3. National Safety Council, *Accident Facts, 1993 Edition* (Itasca, IL: National Safety Council, 1993): 4–5.
4. U.S. Department of Health and Human Services, *Healthy People 2000: National Health Promotion and Disease Prevention Objectives* (Washington, DC: U.S. Government Printing Office, 1991): 280.
5. Ibid.
6. National Safety Council, *Accident Facts 1993,* 103.
7. Jame A. Gulaid and others, "Household Survey of Child-Safe Packaging for Medications," *Public Health Reports* 105, no. 4 (July–August 1990): 430–32.
8. U.S. Department of Health and Human Services, *Healthy People 2000,* 280.

9. Ibid.
10. "Poisoning Hotlines," *Emergency Medicine* 24, no. 2 (15 February 1992): 212–23.
11. *Emergency Medicine,* 249 W. 17th St., New York, NY 10011.
12. Centers for Disease Control and Prevention, *Morbidity and Mortality Weekly Report* 41, no. RR-6 (24 April 1992): 12.
13. Consumer Product Safety Commission document on *Toy Safety,* released November 1990.
14. Ibid.
15. Ibid.

CHAPTER 4

Fire—a Positive and a Negative Force

Chapter Outline

Introduction
What Is Fire?
Classifications of Fires
   Class A Fire
   Class B Fire
   Class C Fire
   Class D Fire
Data Regarding Fires
   Risk Factors
Types of Injuries Related to Fire
   Degree of Burn
   Scalding
   Other Fire-Related Hazards
   Medical Procedures for Burns

Early Warning Systems
   Types of Systems
   Location of the Systems
   Mandatory Regulations
Extinguishing Fires
   Portable Fire Extinguishers
   Community Fire-Fighting Systems
Fire Protection and Prevention
Summary
Discussion Questions
Suggested Readings
Endnotes

Introduction

Fire is one of the great paradoxes in the world. It plays an important role in keeping people warm and comfortable; it is a source of energy; food is prepared over the warmth of a fire. Yet, pain, injury, and death may be inflicted on anyone who comes into contact with fire. The beauty and peacefulness of a campfire or a fire burning in the family room fireplace is something most of us enjoy. A spark from that same campfire or an accidentally deposited cigarette can initiate a forest fire that can cause the destruction of thousands of acres of woodlands, resulting in thousands of dollars of damage and the loss of hundreds of helpless animals as well as human lives. Fire is necessary to many industrial processes. Thousands of degrees of heat are used to manufacture steel and many other products. On the other hand, everything for which a person has worked and saved can be destroyed in a matter of minutes when a house or apartment goes up in flames.

People have long used fire. Early humans learned of the usefulness of fire to clear vegetation so that the land could be cultivated. This procedure, known as "slash and burn," is still used today in many parts of the world. Not only is the land effectively cleared for planting but the ash from this burning process serves as nourishment for the soil.

Fire has been used throughout history for cooking and warmth. Without heat generated by fire, it would be very difficult for people to survive in the coldest regions of the world.

The earliest incidences of fire were no doubt natural. Certainly early humans must have been exposed to fire resulting from the strike of lightning or from volcanic lava. But for many years there probably was no known procedure for starting a fire. Hence, it was necessary to keep a fire burning by adding leaves, twigs, or other combustible material or to carry the burning embers to another location where fire was desired. A breakthrough occurred when people learned how to produce a fire without depending upon nature.

What Is Fire?

Fire is the result of a chemical reaction in which heat and light are produced. Rapid oxidation, combined with some fuel, causes fire. This chemical process is known as *combustion*. The necessary oxidizer in fires is usually oxygen. Flame and heat may be produced without oxygen, as in the case of combining sodium and chlorine, but only when oxygen functions as an oxidizer is the process referred to as "fire." For there to be a fire, three elements must be present: oxygen, fuel, and heat.

In order to extinguish a fire, one of the three necessary elements must be removed. For example, if something is burning and the source of oxygen is removed by smothering the flame, the fire is extinguished. Most of us have put a small burning candle in a glass jar and placed a cover over the top. The flame goes out when the supply of oxygen is cut off.

Because heat is necessary to the production of fire, removal of heat can be used to cool the blaze to a point below the ignition temperature. The temperature at which a substance begins to burn (ignites) will vary. The ignition temperature of a solid material is higher than is that of a liquid, for example. The best means of reducing the temperature of many fires is to apply water. Water will absorb the heat and in the process extinguish the fire.

Two important components of fires are smoke and flame. Flame is the luminous part of the fire that most of us associate with a blaze. A burning building with high shooting flames will attract attention. But a fire may not always have a flame. If there is little oxygen, for example, there is not likely to be a flame. A field of dry grass burning high in the mountains will have little flame because of the absence of oxygen at high elevations.

There is always visible smoke from any kind of fire. Smoke is made up of gaseous products that result from the burning of organic materials. Smoke is not only destructive at the scene of the fire, but it may be blown some distance and cause additional damage. More injuries and deaths occur from smoke inhalation than from exposure to the heat and the flames generated by a fire. As the result of inhaling smoke, an individual becomes asphyxiated because the body cells do not receive the needed oxygen.

Classifications of Fires

Even though most people think of fires as essentially identical, it is important to understand that there are several different types of fires. The particular classification of fire is based upon what objects are burning—which, in turn, impacts the measures needed to be taken to combat the fire. Even though we normally think that spraying water on a fire will effectively extinguish the blaze, there are certain kinds of fire for which such measures are ineffective and actually may serve to spread the fire. Four different classifications of fire have been identified.

Class A Fire

Class A fires are the type with which most individuals are familiar. This type of fire occurs when ordinary combustible material such as paper, wood, rubbish, clothing, and a variety of other objects are set ablaze. Any substance that burns and leaves an ash is a Class A fire. The principle measure for extinguishing this type of fire is to deny heat in order

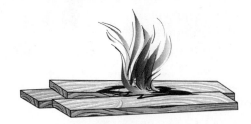

Class A Fire—A fire involving combustible materials such as wood, paper, cloth, and blankets.

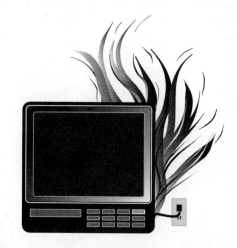

Class C Fire—A fire involving a malfunctioning electrical appliance or caused by faulty wiring.

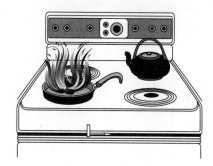

Class B Fire—A fire involving flammable liquids or greases, such as in a frying pan on the stove.

to bring the temperature below the ignition level. This is accomplished most commonly by pouring water on the fire, which cools the fire and prohibits the blaze from spreading.

Class B Fire

Fires that involve the burning of flammable liquids are Class B fires. This type of fire includes the burning of such products as grease, oil, gasoline, and kerosene. Fires of this type usually spread rapidly. It is necessary when confronted with a Class B fire to cut off oxygen from the blaze. This is accomplished by smothering the fire, often with foam. It is unwise to use water in attempts to extinguish this type of fire. A stream of water may actually cause the flaming liquid to splash and contribute to the spread of the blaze.

Class C Fire

Electrical fires are Class C fires. These fires result from shorts in electrical lines and from the overloading of electrical lines and outlets. The energy running through the electrical lines and/or appliances become overheated and a fire results.

Water should not be used in attempts to put out electrical fires because water is a good conductor of electricity. The electrical current can travel through the water and cause serious injury to those attempting to put out the fire. It is important to cut the flow of electrical current at the site of the blaze. However, Class C fires may be extinguished with a fire extinguisher without turning the power off.

Class D Fire

Class D is a classification applied to fires of combustible metals such as potassium, titanium, sodium, and magnesium. These kinds of fires are more commonly found in industrial settings than in homes, schools, and public buildings. It is necessary in combatting this type of fire to isolate the blaze and keep it from spreading. Class D fires require special extinguishing agents that smother the fire and cut off the source of oxygen.

Data Regarding Fires

Injuries from fires are the fifth leading cause of unintentional-injury deaths in the United States. It is estimated that fires cause more than 4,000 fatalities a year.[1] Eighty-five percent of these deaths are the result of fires occurring in the home. Two-thirds of the fire-related fatalities are caused by exposure to toxic gases, actually resulting in suffocation from lack of adequate oxygen. About one-fourth of the fatalities are the result of burns over various parts of the body.

In addition, more than 105,000 disabling injuries a year are caused by fire with more than a million burn injuries a year requiring some medical attention. Many individuals requiring hospitalization suffer injuries that result in permanent scarring and disfigurement.

The economic cost of unintentional injuries that occur from fires is estimated to run as high as ten billion dollars annually. In addition to medical costs and lost production, there are also property damages including loss of the structure which may be destroyed completely as well as the contents of the building. Other losses are less tangible. Many times items of value destroyed in home and office fires cannot have a monetary value placed on them because they are irreplaceable.

Fires resulting in injury and death occur at all times of the year, though the peak mortality period is in the winter months—with January being the highest. This is because heating equipment such as furnaces, electric heaters, and stoves are in greatest use during this time. Every effort should be made to assure that any heating device is properly maintained.

Fatalities and injuries due to fires are most common among the elderly and the very young, as these population groups are the least likely to be able to help themselves when caught in a burning building. Unfortunately, rarely does a winter pass when there are not reports of a nursing home fire involving several fatalities. Many reasons can be cited for these occurrences. In some localities, strong fire ordinances are lacking for nursing homes. Also, when fire does occur in a nursing home, there often is a serious lack of personnel available to assist the removal of the elderly from the burning building. Since many of these individuals are invalids and cannot escape on their own, fatality all too often results.

The importance of reducing fatalities from fires, particularly residential fires, was noted in the national health promotion and disease prevention objectives for the year 2000.[2] A measurable objective, as published in that 1990 initiative, is to achieve a fatality rate reduction from 1.5 to 1.2 per 100,000 by the year 2000. In order to obtain this fatality rate, four population groups have been targeted for particular program emphasis: children four years of age and younger, senior citizens, African-American males, and African-American females. African-Americans account for over 15 percent of all deaths due to fire-related injuries. The death rate for African-American males is three times the rate for white males and five times the rate of white females. There are several possible reasons for this. Poor housing with lack of early warning detectors and inappropriate heating devices are two major reasons. Also, there is greater incidence of fires starting as the result of smoking cigarettes in bed among African-American males than other population groups.

Risk Factors

Although many behavioral risk factors contribute to fires, three merit consideration: use of alcohol, smoking, and activities associated with the use of matches and cigarette lighters.

Alcohol use is a major factor impacting the number of residential fires. Individuals who are intoxicated often fall asleep while smoking in bed. In nearly half of all fire fatalities, the individual is legally drunk at the time of the occurrence. The most probable risk factor associated with alcohol use and fire and burn injuries is cigarette smoking.

Intoxication also may prevent one from hearing a fire alarm—hence, prevent one from taking measures to escape the burning building. Alcoholic intoxication affects judgment and inhibits an individual's responses and reflexes, further hampering the ability to escape from the fire.

There is some evidence that alcohol acts synergistically with toxic gases such as carbon monoxide in accelerating behavioral incapacitation.[3] Also, people with serious burns who have a history of alcohol abuse may be at greater risk of succumbing to injuries. There is some evidence of a clinical basis for this. Alcoholism can impair liver function, and liver plays a role in assisting the body to recover from burns.[4]

Smoking is another major risk factor in residential dwelling fires—particularly smoking while in bed or lying on a couch. In the likelihood of an individual falling asleep, a fire can very quickly begin.

Abandoned cigarettes are another very common cause of fire. Ashes from cigarettes may lodge in upholstered furniture, the sofa, mattress, or bedding and smolder for some time. It is important to check the pieces of furniture on which a smoker has been sitting. Ashtrays should be available and used by those individuals who are smoking. When emptying an ashtray, all cigarette butts and ashes need to be extinguished.

Every year several thousand people require hospital emergency room treatment for injuries associated with matches, lighters, and lighter fluid. Children, in particular, are burned and injured as the result of playing with these items.

Most people know basic fire safety rules that we should close a matchbox cover before striking a match, that matchbooks with the striking surface on the back should be used, and that children should be taught the dangers of playing with matches. Yet many costly fires occur from the failure to follow these simple procedures.

The Consumer Product Safety Commission has developed a standard that requires matchbooks to be "childproof." Every matchbook is required to have a latch that makes it difficult, if not impossible, for children to open. Basically the latch requires two separate motions to open. It is felt that such a latch will prohibit many injuries, particularly to small children.

Types of Injuries Related to Fire

Burns are tissue injuries caused most commonly by fire. Injury to the tissue stems from exposure to heat. However, fire is not the only agent that can cause burn tissue injuries. Electrical current, chemicals, hot liquid or steam, explosion, and radiation can all damage tissue.

Degree of Burn

The most familiar aspect of burn injury is damage to the skin, a damage that is identified in terms of the degree of destruction. A *first-degree burn* is a shallow injury characterized by a reddening of the skin. A scald resulting from exposure to hot water or steam is a common example. This type of burn is often observed after an individual has spent several hours sunbathing on the beach.

A burn which results in a deepened extent of damage to the skin is a *second-degree burn,* although the entire skin layer is not affected. Usually this degree of burn is distinguishable by the presence of blisters.

When the entire layer of skin is affected, it is referred to as a *third-degree burn.* This type of burn will normally result in the destruction of the skin and possibly the underlying structures. Charring of tissue may result. Third-degree burns often result in a loss of body fluid, which leads to shock. Hemorrhaging and the consequent blood loss complicate these types of burn injuries.

Scalding

Scalds result from exposure to moist heat, hot water, and steam. Exposure to hot water exceeding 130 degrees Fahrenheit can cause serious injury with as little as two to three seconds of exposure. Usually scalding results in second- and third-degree injuries. The Centers for Disease Control and Prevention recommended at the National Injury Control Conference in 1992 that settings on hot water heaters should be set at no higher than 120 degrees Fahrenheit.[5]

Many preventive measures can be taken to reduce the possibility of scalds. If water from the hot water tap is too hot to the touch, the thermostat on the hot water heater should be lowered. Always test the bath water temperature before getting into the bathtub. This practice is most important prior to placing a small child into the tub.

Other Fire-Related Hazards

One of the basic purposes that the skin serves is to protect the internal body structures from microorganisms that cause infection. Whenever there is a break in the skin, the possibility for infection is greatly increased. Since there is skin damage associated with both second- and third-degree burns, the likelihood of infection is a matter demanding immediate attention. Treatment of infection often becomes the most difficult and serious problem in many burn cases.

Possibly as many as two-thirds of all fatalities from fires are due to inhalation of gases caused by the blaze. Most victims of a fire do not burn to death; they die from carbon monoxide poisoning—asphyxiation. Toxic gases are generated by the blaze. Exposure to carbon monoxide and other gases may cause enough lung damage to impede normal respiratory functioning. When a person falls asleep while smoking, the victim is often unaware of the blaze, and death occurs from carbon monoxide poisoning.

Burning materials containing various chemicals can cause serious injury and death. For example, polyvinyl chloride (PVC) is a common component used in various home construction materials. It is found in electrical and telephone wiring insulation where it serves as a substitute for rubber. Burning PVC presents special hazards involving inhalation of vapors. Hydrogen chloride, inhaled or combined with water vapor, acts as an irritant to the mucous membranes and is particularly dangerous to the respiratory tract and eyes. Irritation of the throat and spasms of the larynx may occur. Respiratory distress may develop immediately upon exposure to the smoke generated from a fire, or it may not appear for a day or two after exposure. The period of time just after the fire is extinguished may not seem to be particularly dangerous, but the smoke and fumes that still fill the air may be very toxic.

Medical Procedures for Burns

The immediate care that should be rendered to an individual who has experienced burn injuries is to immerse the burned area for a period of time, between 10 to 15 minutes, in cold water. This procedure will cool the heat associated with the fire. It also helps to reduce pain and the possibility of greater depth of burn injury.

Note that water should not be applied directly on an open burn of the skin. Instead, it is recommended that the area be covered with a thick clean cloth and then cooled with a bag or bottle of cold water.

Numerous other inappropriate emergency care procedures are practiced by some people. Probably the most commonly practiced measure that is of no value is the application of butter to the burn. This practice has no value in treating the burn and may result in contamination to the tissues.

Medical burn treatment may be long-term and expensive. The victim often faces psychological and emotional problems, in addition to physical injuries, because of the scarring and physical disability that may accompany a burn. Medical treatment of the injured person involves more than treating the patient. The family or close associates of the injured often are affected emotionally by the injuries. Such a reaction may stem from personal feelings for the injured individual or from a psychological reaction at having witnessed the result of the trauma—sight of the burn itself, presence of blood, and associated tissue damage.

Early Warning Systems

Early fire warning devices play an important role in reducing the likelihood of injury to people from fires. Such devices in the home have played a significant role in reducing residential fire injuries in the past decade. Today, approximately three out of every four homes have at least one early warning detector. The percentage of residential dwellings having early fire detection devices increased significantly during the 1980s. Several reasons could be given for the increase in the installation and use of these systems during the past decade. Public awareness of the usefulness of the early warning detection devices in giving early warning of a fire has increased their purchase and use. In some localities legislation and regulations have been mandated, requiring installation of detectors in homes. The cost of such devices is reasonable, so that expense should not be a factor keeping most individuals from installing them.

The importance of smoke detectors in all residential dwellings has been recognized by the federal government health objectives initiative for the year 2000.[6] An objective proposes having at least one functional smoke detector on each floor of all dwellings by the year 2000. To achieve this objective, such devices will need to become the norm in an additional one out of every four residential dwellings.

Types of Systems

Two different types of early warning systems are on the market today. One is a smoke detector, and the other, a sensory detector.

Smoke Detector

Smoke detectors work on the principle that shortly after a blaze ignites, smoke from the fire can be detected and an early warning signal given. Since most fatalities from a fire result from smoke inhalation and because smoke spreads faster than heat, a smoke detector can give a warning before the smoke has built up to a dangerous level.

There are two kinds of smoke detectors: the photoelectric detector and the ion chamber detector. The photoelectric detector senses a smoldering fire more quickly than it does a flaming fire. The device works on the light scattering principle. A photoelectric bulb emits a beam of light that sets up an electric current in the detector. When smoke obscures this photoelectric light, the flow of current to the detector is reduced and the alarm is activated. This detector responds more readily to light, visible smoke.

The ion chamber detector operates on a slightly different principle. Key components are two inner chambers and a radioactive source. Rays from the source flow into the sensing chamber, and any particle entering the chamber changes the balance of voltage and triggers the alarm. The process by which the alarm is sounded depends on a complex electrical reaction involving the radiation source and molecules (ions) in the air at the point a fire originates. This type of detector is more sensitive than the photoelectric detector in "sensing" fire at the earliest stages.

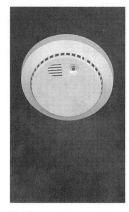

Early warning systems are now required by public regulations in many communities.

Sensory Detector

A second type of early warning fire detection makes use of heat sensing. The heat sensor activates an alarm system when a certain temperature level is reached. This system will indicate when a fire is burning in the area where the sensor is located. Most fire prevention agencies suggest that these systems be placed in kitchens, garages, attics, basements, and rooms with fireplaces. It is in these areas of the home that blazing fires are most likely to start. The heat sensor detection system is of little use in the bedroom areas of the house. By the time the fire has reached a level that will activate this system, it is too late for the sleeping person to escape.

There also are flame detector systems that sense light from the flames. When a flame is present, the alarm system will go off. By the time a fire is at this stage, it has probably destroyed much property, and the value of such a system in a home is questionable.

Automatic Sprinklers

Though not found as often in homes, apartments, and other residential dwellings, automatic sprinklers are required in many public buildings. For example, in most hotels and motels, theaters, and other buildings where large crowds gather, it is mandatory that there be automatic sprinkler systems. There are some local ordinances that require the installation of residential sprinklers in multiple-family residential dwellings.

The most commonly found sprinkler system is the wet pipe system. In this system the pipes are full of water under pressure. The sprinkler head is activated by a small heat detector and water is discharged. In areas where freezing pipes can be a problem, a dry pipe

Fire—a Positive and a Negative Force

system is employed. With this system the pipes are filled with dry compressed air. When activated, there is a slight delay before water reaches the fire.

Location of the Systems

In residential dwellings early warning smoke detectors should be placed near or on the ceiling. One of the best locations is at the top of a stairway. Also, it is wise to place the device near the bedroom area of the house. This will provide an early warning safety valve while the residents in the house are asleep. Most fire safety agencies recommend that a smoke detector also be placed in the basement.

It is important that maintenance of the early warning detection system be carried out on a regular basis. Most systems operate on batteries. Should the batteries not be functioning properly, the usefulness of the system is of no value. It has been reported that two-thirds of all detector system failures during fire are the result of dead batteries.[7] Every detector should be checked for proper operation at least on a monthly basis. Hold a lighted candle about six inches from the detector. If the alarm fails to go off, it is not working properly.

Mandatory Regulations

Many local and state regulations have been implemented in recent years mandating the installation of early warning detection systems in residential dwellings. Some regulations mandate that alarm systems must be included in all new building construction, including houses. Others now require that apartments, regardless of age, must have such warning devices. Because of the inexpensive nature of smoke detectors, it seems logical to suggest that the goal of having such detection devices in every residential dwelling by the year 2000 should be achieved prior to that time. In an attempt to assist certain economically-disadvantaged individuals, it has been reported that one community was making smoke detectors available at no cost to those in need.[8]

Extinguishing Fires

As important as it is for each of us to take measures to prevent fires from happening, serious life-threatening and property-destroying fires do occur. It is therefore important that measures be instituted to extinguish the blaze. How this is accomplished will be determined somewhat by what type of fire is burning, by what fire-fighting equipment is available, and the skills of those available to use the equipment.

Portable Fire Extinguishers

Portable fire extinguishers are valuable in putting out small fires before they have the opportunity to grow into a major blaze. These extinguishers are particularly valuable for home use. There should be at least one, and preferably more, portable fire extinguishers in every residential dwelling. The building occupants must know how to use the extinguisher and should be assured that they are in proper operating condition.

There are different types of fire extinguishers designed to counter different classifications of fire. Home-use extinguishers usually contain one of three dry chemicals: sodium bicarbonate, potassium bicarbonate, and ammonium phosphate. Only ammonium phosphate is effective against Class A, Class B, and Class C fires. The kind of fire against which any given extinguisher is to be used is noted on the label.

In addition to the class of fire indicated by the *letter,* the label should also indicate by *number* the appropriate size of fire that can be extinguished. The code begins with the number one for a small fire—a code system that increases as the potential fire size increases. For example, an extinguisher labeled 10-B is more effective than one rated 2-B.

When purchasing a fire extinguisher, be sure that it will be effective for the kind of fire most likely to occur in the area where it is to be kept. For example, around kitchens, fires will generally result from grease or electrical appliances. A fire extinguisher with a B:C rating should be available in this location. Since in bedrooms fires may stem from combustible material such as clothing or bedding, an extinguisher designed to be used with Class A fires should be available. All fire extinguishers should be kept near a doorway, but out of reach of children.

Fire extinguishers are relatively easy to operate. Yet everyone who has one should take active measures to learn how it operates *before* a fire occurs, as operating mechanisms do vary from one extinguisher to another. There will be no time for instruction reading once a fire has begun. In operation of the extinguisher, aim the contents at the base of the fire, not at the flames or the smoke, and use a sweeping, side-to-side motion.

It is important to know when to use a fire extinguisher. Fire-fighting personnel advise that an individual should always call the fire department before attempting to fight the fire with a fire extinguisher. If an individual uses the extinguisher without calling the fire department and then the fire is not extinguished, precious time has been lost. Obviously the ideal situation is to have one person call the fire department while another is using the fire extinguisher.

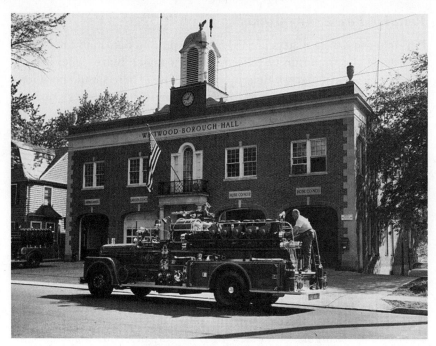

The fire engine is the basic fire-fighting equipment used in communities with full-time fire-fighting personnel, as well as those with volunteer fire departments.

Community Fire-Fighting Systems

Throughout the United States, fire-fighting services are maintained by cities, towns, communities, and other political jurisdictions. Most urban cities have fire departments that employ professional, trained fire-fighting personnel. These individuals are employed as full-time fire-fighters with funding for operation of this service coming from taxation.

Small communities and rural townships have volunteer fire-fighting personnel. These individuals are employed full-time in various lines of work and have received training in fire-fighting techniques and procedures. When a fire occurs, an alarm system summons the volunteer members to the fire. These systems are necessary particularly in localities where there are not adequate financial resources to employ full-time fire-fighting personnel.

The basic fire-fighting apparatus is the "fire engine," a pumper that takes water by suction and propels it under pressure through fire hoses. In cities that have high-rise buildings, hydraulically operated extension ladder systems make it possible to combat fires several stories above ground level. Fireboats, which are able to pump water onto a fire along a waterway, are especially useful when industrial sites, warehouses, and oil storage facilities are located on the edge of a canal, river, or lake.

The preparation and training of professional fire-fighting personnel, whether full-time or volunteer, is always being upgraded. There are numerous categories of skill that the firefighter is expected to achieve. As fire fighting becomes more technical, the training of fire-fighting personnel is more specialized. For this reason many fire-fighting personnel may enroll in colleges with programs of fire science designed to make them more effective.

There are ongoing initiatives designed to improve the protective equipment available to fire fighters. Particular interest has centered on the development of lighter, yet more superior fire-fighting equipment and clothing. For example, most fire fighters now have personal alert safety systems. These electronic devices, worn by the fire fighter, emit a loud sound anytime the individual doesn't move for over a thirty-second period of time. This helps to locate any fire fighter working in a smoke-filled room who has been overcome by the smoke and fumes. Another piece of equipment that is helpful to fire fighters is the pressure ventilator. The ventilator is placed inside a burning building to blow smoke out of the way so that the fire fighters are able to see more clearly.

In addition to their responsibilities in extinguishing fires, fire fighters also deliver other services in many communities. They often are qualified to deliver emergency medical services, as well as to cope with hazardous materials spills. Fire fighting is obviously one of the more dangerous occupations in the United States. In addition to problems associated with the blaze itself, the firefighter is exposed to various toxic gases, to carcinogens, and other hazardous chemicals. Annually more than one hundred firefighters are killed in the line of duty. Also more than 100,000 firefighters are injured each year while fighting fires.

Fire Protection and Prevention

Measures need to be taken to inform people what to do in case of a fire. Also, every individual should learn how to practice measures that will prevent the occurrence of a fire. This is true whether at one's place of employment, in public settings in the community, or at home. Of particular concern are measures that need to be taken to improve fire safety around the home.

The National Fire Protection Association has suggested several strategies to reduce potential fire hazards at home:[9]

1. All possible fire hazards should be removed or corrected.
2. Every family member should be taught fire prevention concepts.

3. Early warning systems need to be a part of each home.
4. Every family member should know what to do in case of fire.

There are any number of potential hazards that can cause a fire to start in a home. It is important that the heating system be checked annually to make sure that it is functioning properly, safely, and efficiently. Chimneys should be kept clean and heating pipe connections should fit snugly.

Proper loading of electrical circuits will help to prevent electrical fires. Electrical repairs or new installations should only be undertaken if an individual knows exactly what to do and how it should be done. Otherwise a licensed electrician should do the work.

Other potentially serious fire hazards are the storage areas around the house. Basements, attics, stairwells, and any other storage area should be kept free of combustible items. For example, greasy or oily rags, paint, and gasoline should not be left where they or their fumes can be ignited easily.

The National Fire Protection Association recommends that every family member be taught fire prevention concepts. All individuals, children as well as adults, should work to establish personal habits that promote fire prevention and fire safety. An increased awareness of fire and how to cope with it will be helpful if these concepts are ever needed.

Another recommendation of the National Fire Protection Association is that every family member should know what to do in case of a fire. Few families have developed a fire escape plan from their house. Yet this is something that every family should do. If all the family members are involved in the development of a home safety plan, there will be greater understanding of how to take action when needed.

At least two exits from each room in the house should be noted and identified. One exit will be the regular door leading from the room. In some rooms, particularly bedrooms, it will mean designating a window that can be opened easily. In a two-story home this may be difficult. If possible, windows selected for exit purposes should open onto porch roofs. The National Fire Protection Association suggests that people keep the bedroom door closed when sleeping. This will help to slow the spread of a fire in the bedroom section of the house.

Some families have fire safety ladders to be used for escape from second-floor bedrooms. Not only should they be universally available, but family members should know how to use them. A family fire drill needs to be conducted occasionally, particularly in homes with small children. Unfortunately, there are few families who take the time to carry out a home fire drill.

FIRE DEPARTMENT TELEPHONE NUMBER

The telephone number of the local fire department in my community is _____.

When a fire occurs, it is important not to leave a room and enter a hallway until there is assurance that it is safe to do so. If there might be a fire on the other side of a closed door, do not open it. An individual should touch the closed door to determine whether or not it is hot. If the door is hot, there is danger in opening it. The blaze in the room or hallway on the other side of the door causes the buildup of dangerous amounts of carbon monoxide. If allowed to rush into the room, this gas—in addition to the superheated atmosphere—may cause instant death upon exposure. Whenever a closed door is hot, look for an alternate escape route from the room.

Heat and smoke tend to rise. If trapped by fire in a building, stay as low to the floor as possible and crawl toward a safe location. Also take measures to protect the lungs and the hair. Hair burns very rapidly and heat can cause serious damage to the lungs. It is wise to place a cloth, towel, or handkerchief over the head and the mouth. If the material is wet, it will be more effective in providing protection.

When trapped in a room with an outside window, open it slightly at the top and the bottom. The trapped individual also should stay in the room if possible. It is important never to jump for safety, except as a last resort.

Should one's clothes catch on fire, it is necessary to immediately take measures to smother the blaze. Rolling on the ground or wrapping a coat or blanket around the victim will help to extinguish flames. A natural reaction in this situation is to run. Running only causes the flames to spread and burn more rapidly.

An education strategy that is taught by fire-fighting personnel to elementary school age children is the *stop-drop-and-roll* technique. This activity teaches children that in cases where their clothing is on fire they should immediately stop and drop to the ground. When on the ground they should roll around to smother the flames. This teaching strategy is very well received by young children and provides them with a clear understanding of what to do when their clothing is burning.

In establishing a home fire escape plan, a prearranged meeting place should be designated outside the house or apartment. This will facilitate knowing if all the occupants of the burning building are out of danger—a particularly valuable procedure for families with a number of children.

One other important matter that seems almost unnecessary to mention is that every person should know, or have written in an obvious location, the telephone number of the local fire department. At the time of a fire, minutes saved are vitally important. Time spent trying to find the phone number of the fire department can result in tragedy.

Summary

Fire can be a source of warmth, heat, and beauty or a roaring inferno sweeping through a high-rise office building causing millions of dollars of property damage and injuring many people. Fire is both necessary and helpful and destructive and fatal. People have had to learn to live with fire and to take important measures to prevent disastrous incidents.

There are many causes of fires. Each year over a million people seek medical care and more than 4,000 fatalities occur as a result of fire. More than 100,000 disabling injuries annually are caused by fire. The home is especially vulnerable to fire.

Fires are divided into four classes: Class A fires involve ordinary combustible material, Class B fires involve flammable liquids, Class C fires are electrical in nature, and Class D fires include combustible metals and normally take place in an industrial setting.

There are many preventive measures that can be taken to protect against the destruction of a fire. Early fire warning detection devices play a major role in reducing the incidence of fire. There are two different types of early warning detection systems: the smoke detector and the sensory detector.

There should be a fire extinguisher in every residential dwelling. Purchasers of fire extinguishers must be certain that they have selected extinguishers that will be effective against the class of fire most likely to occur in their environment. Not only is it important to have the proper kind of extinguisher, but people must know how to operate such devices before the occurrence of a fire.

Fire fighting is an important occupation in our society. Most communities have some kind of fire-fighting organization. Different kinds of equipment and training go into the development of an individual fire-fighting system. It is important that increasing research and training be implemented to improve the quality of community fire-fighting equipment and personnel.

Because of the potential hazards associated with home fires, each family should develop a fire safety plan. Plans should be established for safe evacuation from any dwelling in time of a fire. Everyone should know the dangers of becoming isolated in a burning building and become familiar with measures necessary to escape safely.

Discussion Questions

1. What occurs chemically when there is a fire?
2. What are the three elements that must be present for there to be a fire?
3. Differentiate the four classes of fire.
4. What are the appropriate measures for extinguishing a Class A and a Class B fire?
5. What objectives have been identified relating to fire in the nation's health initiative for the year 2000?
6. Why is alcohol considered to be a risk factor associated with fires?
7. Differentiate between a first-, second-, and third-degree burn.
8. Explain the difference between a smoke and fire detector.
9. Explain the principle underlying operation of the ion chamber detector.
10. What are appropriate locations in a residential dwelling for fire detectors?
11. What are some procedures that can be taken by a family in reducing the potential fire hazards around the home?
12. What measures should be taken to extinguish the flames when one's clothing is on fire?

Suggested Readings

Bill, Robert G., and Kung Hsiang-Cheng. "Limited-Water-Supply Sprinklers for Manufactured (Mobile) Homes," *Fire Technology* 29, no. 3 (March 1993): 203–25.

Black, Carla F. "Preventing Fire in the Home," *Consumers' Research* 73, no. 12 (December 1990): 10–14.

Centers for Disease Control and Prevention. "Position Papers from the Third National Injury Control Conference: Setting the National Agenda for Injury Control in the 1990s, Fire- and Burn-Related Injuries," *Morbidity and Mortality Weekly Report* 41, no. RR-6 (24 April 1992): 13–14.

Council on Scientific Affairs. "Preventing Death and Injury from Fires with Automatic Sprinklers and Smoke Detectors," *Journal of the American Medical Association* 257 (27 March 1987): 1618–20.

Gulaid, Jame A., Richard W. Sattin, and Richard J. Waxweiler. "Deaths From Residential Fires, 1978–1984," *Morbidity and Mortality Weekly Report* 37, no. SS-1 (February 1988): 39–45.

Gulaid, Jame A., and others. "Differences in Death Rates Due to Injury Among Blacks and Whites, 1984," *Morbidity and Mortality Weekly Report* 37, no. SS-3 (July 1988): 25–31.

Hall, John R. *The United States Fire Problem Overview Report Through 1990: Leading Causes and Other Patterns and Trends.* Quincy, MA: National Fire Protection Association, 1992.

Howland, Jonathan, and Ralph Hingson. "Alcohol as a Risk Factor for Injuries or Death Due to Fires and Burns: Review of the Literature," *Public Health Reports* 102, no. 5 (September–October 1987): 475–83.

National Fire Protection Association. *Standard for the Installation of Sprinkler Systems in One- and Two- Family Dwellings and Mobile Homes.* Quincy, MA: National Fire Protection Association, 1980.

Planek, Thomas W. "Home Accidents: A Continuing Social Problem," *Accident Analysis and Prevention,* 14, no. 2 (February 1982): 107–20.

Randall, Jeff, and Russell T. Jones. "Teaching Children Fire Safety Skills," *Fire Technology* 29, no. 3 (March 1993): 268–80.

Runyon, Carol W., and others. "Risk Factors for Fatal Residential Fires," *Fire Technology* 29, no. 2 (February 1993): 183–93.

Shaw, Kathy N., and others. "Correlates of Reported Smoke Detector Usage in an Inner-City Population: Participants in a Smoke Detector Give-Away Program." *American Journal of Public Health* 78, no. 6 (June 1988): 650–53.

Shults, J. D. " Proper Storage Stops Fires," *Safety and Health* 145, no. 2 (February 1992): 46–48.

Walker, Bonnie L., and others. "The Short-Term Effects of a Fire Safety Education Program for the Elderly," *Fire Technology* 28, no. 2 (May 1992): 134–62.

In addition, a variety of useful materials relating to fire safety are prepared and available from: National Fire Protection Association, Batterymarch Park, Quincy, MA 02269.

Endnotes

1. Data presented in this section are from National Safety Council, *Accident Facts, 1993 Edition* (Chicago, IL: National Safety Council 1993), 4.
2. U.S. Department of Health and Human Services, Public Health Service, *Healthy People 2000: National Health Promotion and Disease Prevention Objectives* (Washington, DC: U.S. Government Printing Office, 1991), 278.
3. Jonathan Howland and Ralph Hingson, "Alcohol as a Risk Factor for Injuries or Death Due to Fires and Burns: Review of the Literature," *Public Health Reports* 102, no. 5 (September–October 1987): 482.
4. Ibid., 481.
5. Centers for Disease Control and Prevention, " Position Papers from the Third National Injury Control Conference: Setting the National Agenda for Injury Control in the 1990s," *Morbidity and Mortality Weekly Report* 41, no. RR-6 (24 April 1992): 14.
6. U.S. Department of Health and Human Services, Public Health Service, *Healthy People 2000*, 285.
7. Ibid.
8. Kathy N. Shaw and others, "Correlates of Reported Smoke Detector Usage in an Inner-City Population: Participants in a Smoke Detector Give-Away Program," *American Journal of Public Health* 78, no. 6 (June 1988): 650–53.
9. Statements attributed in this section to the National Fire Protection Association are from various public information releases and brochures of the National Fire Protection Association, Batterymarch Park, Quincy, MA 02269.

CHAPTER 5

Safety in the Workplace—Economic as Well as Personal Concerns

Chapter Outline

Introduction
Workplace Safety Data
History of Occupational Safety
Occupational Safety and Health Act of 1970
  Purpose of the Legislation
  Areas of Mandated Activity
  Relationship of OSHA with the States
  Impact of OSHA
Occupational Safety Objectives for the Year 2000
Personnel Involved in Occupational Safety
  Industrial Hygienists
  Safety Engineers
  Occupational Physicians and Nurses

Selected Work Sites
  Mining
  Transportation
Employee Occupational Safety Initiatives
  Personal Protective Equipment
  Employee Motivational Programs
Summary
Discussion Questions
Suggested Readings
Endnotes

Introduction

Everyone reading this chapter is currently employed, or upon completion of an education program, will find work opportunities. For some it may mean self-employment, working out of one's home, or at a location with a small number of other employees. For others, it may be employment with a multinational corporation employing thousands of individuals. Whatever the size of workplace and location of employment, a safe work environment is important. The safety of one's place of employment is predicated upon many factors. Daily, individuals are exposed to many situations that can be dangerous to the personal safety and well-being of the employee. One's well-being, both personal and economic, is impacted by how safe a person is from injury associated with the workplace.

Workplace Safety Data

The federal government estimates that there are more than 110 million persons in the American workplace.[1] It is difficult, however, to get an accurate statistical picture of the extent of work-related fatalities and injuries. This is due to the fact that most statistical reporting of occupational-related fatalities and injuries is based on analysis of inferential data. This means that data are obtained by taking random sampling of the population. Accuracy is difficult because different sampling techniques are used by the various agencies which usually report statistics. There are also differences in definitions of what constitutes a work fatality, a work-related injury, or a disabling injury.

The problem of obtaining exact data on work-related fatalities and injuries is demonstrated by the fact that for a recent year the number of fatalities reported in work-related circumstances ranged from 3,000 to nearly 11,000.[2] It is obvious that there is a need for a more reliable count of all work-related fatalities. In order to accomplish this the Bureau of Labor Statistics has designed a process known as a Census of Fatal Occupational Injuries. This Census, initially tested in cooperation with the Texas Department of Health, includes information about age, occupation, and other demographic data associated with all work-related fatalities.[3] It is planned that the process will be implemented in all states by the mid-1990s and that a national database will be established to provide accurate data on workplace-related fatalities and injuries.

The National Safety Council, which issues reports annually using their inferential database, has stated that approximately 8,500 lives are lost annually in work-related occurrences.[4] It was also reported that

3.3 million disabling injuries occurred in the occupational setting. A disabling injury is defined by the National Safety Council as an accident in which the injured party is affected beyond the given day of the accident.[5]

In addition to fatality- and injury-related issues, other factors are relevant. Lost work time results from injury-producing situations that occur on the job, involving one or more days of absence from work. It is estimated that over 65 million workdays are lost each year as the result of work-related accidents. Two-thirds of these result in a loss of more than seven days of work. Not only is this loss relevant for the present, but usually the time loss affects the future production and performance of the individual on the job. The National Safety Council projected in 1993 that time loss in future years from accidents which occurred in 1992 would be nearly 110 million workdays.[6]

Economic factors of accident-related work injuries are dimensions often overlooked when thinking about workplace safety. In order to remain viable any business and industry must yield a profit. If costs and lost work time are affected to a significant degree by injuries, the profitability of American businesses is negatively affected. The estimated cost of work-related accidents in a recent year was $115.9 billion.[7] This included wages lost, medical expenses, insurance costs, fire losses, and taxes not paid on earned wages including social security taxes. Expenses are not only related to the worker. Accidents often result in damage to equipment that must be repaired or replaced as well as shutdown time on the assembly line in a factory.

The majority of work-related fatalities and injuries are preventable. Training the employee in proper safety procedures which lead to safe practices can effectively reduce such occurrences. Engineering safety in the workplace environment is possibly the best approach to reducing the number of work-related fatalities and serious injuries. The provision and use of protective equipment also can help to protect against work-related fatalities and injuries.

History of Occupational Safety

During the early Colonial years in the United States most people lived in rural settings, worked the land, and provided for much of their own economic needs. The major focus of life centered around farming and tasks related to carving a society out of the wilderness.

Individuals lived in small houses and farmed the land on which they lived. Many of the tools and equipment used in those early days were rather simple when compared with the sophisticated machinery

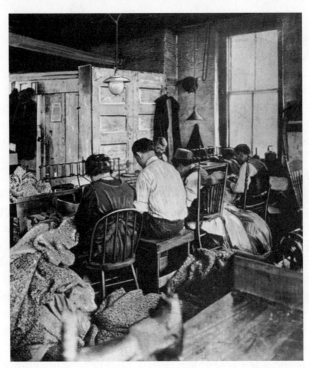

Conditions in the workplace have improved greatly since the 1800s. However, it is still necessary to implement measures to continue to provide as safe a workplace as is possible.

found on the farm and in industry today. Though injury- and fatality-producing accidents occurred, they were not widespread. Only as the nation became more urbanized and industrialized did concern for problems associated with occupational accidents—including their causes and prevention—become an area of serious research and study.

During the latter years of the 1800s the United States moved from an agricultural to an industrial society. Industrial development during this period was rapid, accompanied by growth in population and urbanization. Working conditions were generally poor. There was very little effort or initiative directed toward improving these conditions. The only real concern for such issues was expressed when injury prohibited individuals from being able to work—that is, when production was affected. Little concern was shown for the individual. When an injury occurred, there were no compensation programs to assist the employee and his or her family, nor was there financial support for the family or workers killed while working. All too often there was a lack of employer concern for the individual worker. If people became injured there was an attitude that they could be replaced and that the productivity of the corporation would continue.

In the early industrial years of the nineteenth century, the two major threats to workers were fire and amputation.[8] Fires occurred in all kinds of occupational settings. There were few laws, ordinances, and regulations that could assure protection against fire. In many industrial settings hand and finger, as well as foot and toe, amputations were common. There were few, if any, mandates for protective shields on mechanized equipment or tools during these years.

The industrial safety movement had its beginning in the last decade of the 1800s when several developments of note took place.[9] In 1894 Underwriters Laboratories, Inc. was founded. The original purpose of this organization was to assure the safety of elevators in the multistory buildings that were being built in Chicago at this time. Fire hazards in general were a major concern. As a result, fire inspections and written safety standards for elevators became an important component of the work of UL. These early initiatives led to improved fire safety in industry and efforts designed to reduce death and injury in the workplace.

Two years later, in 1896, the National Fire Protection Association was founded. This organization has since become a leader in fire prevention research, technological development, and programming. The activities of this agency have had significant positive effects upon fire prevention in industrial, public, school, and home settings.

At about this same time, the first organized industrial safety program took place at the Illinois Steel Company. It was the steel industry that ''set the pace in safety through the early 1900s.''[10]

During the early years of the twentieth century several important influences on industrial safety developed. In 1911 a worker's compensation law was passed in Wisconsin, the first state to have an effective legal worker's compensation provision. Previously, the states of New York and Maryland had passed such laws, but they had been ruled to be unconstitutional—despite the fact that in 1908 the federal government itself had made a form of worker's compensation available to government employees.

Today every state has a worker's compensation law. Although specific provisions vary, the laws all provide for assistance to those who become injured while on the job. Expenditures for medical and hospital services, for rehabilitation services, and for income compensation are benefits usually available. There is much variation from one state to another in maximum benefit coverage, with each state setting its own level of benefits.

Prior to the 1980s almost all worker's compensation benefits focused on physical injury and illness.[11] However, during the past decade the definition of a ''work-related disability'' has been broadened to include stress-related disorders. For example, mental stress is now considered an occupational disease to be covered by worker's compensation.

The costs of worker's compensation insurance have risen sharply during the past decade. Much of this increase is associated with escalating health care costs. According to the Social Security Administration, compensation paid in a recent year to all workers under worker's compensation laws was approximately $38.2 billion.[12]

In 1912 the Association of Iron and Steel Electrical Engineers held a conference on the problem of accidents, particularly in the workplace, called the First Cooperative Safety Congress. Several other industries were represented at this meeting. Out of this gathering a small organization was formed with the goal of promoting safety—the National Council for Industrial Safety. It opened an office in 1913 in Chicago, but it soon became obvious that safety and accident prevention was important in settings other than industry. For this reason the National Council for Industrial Safety became known as the National Safety Council, enlarged to include safety programming in all areas of life.

The involvement of the federal government in industrial safety began with the establishment of a federal government Department of Labor in 1912. Through the years this department has had a major influence on job safety in the United States.

Much of the early emphasis of occupational safety was on protecting the workplace. With the development of assembly-line production came a new series of problems. Hazards became more complicated and more numerous. An accident on the assembly line could affect not just the injured individual, but possibly the working environment of many others.

By the mid-twentieth century large companies and industries were likely to have some type of safety program. However, most smaller companies had none or they were ineffective. Accident reporting was often voluntary and lacking in uniformity. Any effective safety program was difficult to evaluate because of differing criteria and reporting systems. In some instances the only visible safety activity was the provision of first aid services at the work site.

At the same time, state safety rules and regulations were developed, but they were weak and ineffective for the most part. The employee had little knowledge of required safety standards. There was little effort to identify employee rights and responsibilities.

Federal legislation passed in 1935 and 1945, the Walsh-Healey Acts, mandated that employers with an annual contract of $10,000 with the federal government were required to make certain safety provisions for their employees. During the 1960s a concerted effort was made to pass some kind of federal legislation to improve the health and safety of employees in the industrial and business world.

Occupational Safety and Health Act of 1970

After lengthy debate and discussions, the United States Congress passed the Occupational Safety and Health Act in 1970. This legislation was considered to be a landmark in the field of occupational safety. It was designed to assure that every working person has as safe and healthful a working environment as possible.

There were a number of safety and health problems and concerns that contributed to the initiative for such legislation. At that time over 14,000 persons a year were losing their lives in job-related accidents and some 2.5 million workers were disabled annually. Such statistics highlighted the need for some efforts to make the work site safer. Also of concern to business and industry, both management and labor, was the fact that thousands of workers were exposed to a variety of substances having detrimental effect on their health following long-term exposure.

The provisions of the Occupational Safety and Health Act of 1970 provided the foundation for the establishment of the Occupational Safety and Health Administration (OSHA), an agency organized within the Department of Labor. OSHA has the major responsibility for implementing the various programs mandated by the legislation.

Another government agency established as the result of this act was the National Institute for Occupational Safety and Health (NIOSH), which is today located within the Centers for Disease Control and Prevention of the Department of Health and Human Services (HHS). The Institute's basic responsibility is to conduct research and establish investigation programs in response to the regulations set forth in the Occupational Safety and Health Act (1970) and the Federal Coal Mine Health Act of 1969. NIOSH cannot intervene directly in the workplace; this is the responsibility and role of OSHA.

The basic purpose of the research conducted by NIOSH is to provide data to OSHA so that appropriate exposure levels for hazardous substances and conditions can be determined for workers. The first document published by NIOSH on January 21, 1972 set forth the recommended standards for occupational exposure to asbestos. Since that time criteria documents have been published for more than a hundred other hazardous agents and associated working conditions.

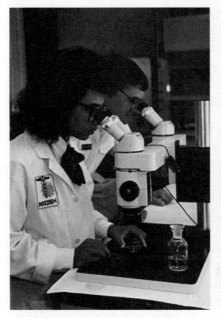 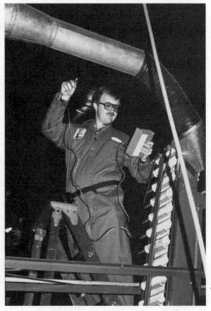

A variety of research is carried out by the National Institute for Occupational Safety and Health. Some research includes examination of microscopic material; other involves use of equipment of various types.

Purpose of the Legislation

Several different factors led to passage of the Occupational Safety and Health Act. The legislation was established primarily to reduce hazards in the workplace for all occupational and industrial employees by establishing mandatory job safety standards. Not only was there a perceived need for standards, but also measures were needed to supervise and enforce such standards, rules, and regulations.

Another purpose of the legislation was to improve accident reporting and record keeping procedures in business and industrial settings. Examination of such data, provided by the Bureau of Labor Statistics, can help to identify job areas and occupational components that are particularly dangerous—hence, warrant the establishment of special accident prevention measures.

In order to establish some common ground for identifying occupational injuries, the legislation defined an *occupational injury* as any disorder that results from an instantaneous exposure. This might be a fall or other direct bodily impact that occurs in the work environment. Disorders that are not instantaneous, but develop over time, are considered to be *workplace-related illnesses*.

Areas of Mandated Activity

Several different types of activities are mandated by the legislation. For our purposes we will discuss four different activities that relate to the Occupational Safety and Health Act: (1) research, (2) establishment of standards, (3) hazard evaluation and inspections, and (4) delineation of employer and employee rights and responsibilities.

Research

Many injuries and fatalities occur each day in workplace settings. The need for and importance of effective research in helping to improve working conditions is treated in certain provisions of the OSHA legislation. Often questions are raised about why and where injuries and fatalities occur. Usually epidemiological studies of specific circumstances will reveal useful information concerning such matters.

Industrial safety research has focused on the psychological, motivational, and behavioral factors relating to accidents on the job. However, more still needs to be learned about why people have accidents in the workplace. Emotional and mental stress have roles to play in causing fatality and injury incidents. Other important questions need answers as well. For example, how can the employee be motivated to use safety equipment without being unduly harassed with rules and regulations? What behavioral factors are commonly associated with employees involved in workplace accidents?

These are examples of questions which research initiatives have attempted to answer. Support for such research activities is authorized and provided under the OSHA legislation. Actual research programs may be carried out by NIOSH, by researchers associated with higher education institutions, at individual research centers, as well as by business and industrial research and development programs.

Establishment of Standards

From research findings come recommendations for the establishment of standards for a safer working environment. Basic premise for such standards is that the place of employment should be as free from as many hazards as possible. Since passage of the legislation, the Occupational Safety and Health Administration (OSHA) has established thousands of standards that apply to millions of working men and women.

Any safety standard established by OSHA must be published in the *Federal Register*. It is then the responsibility of an employer to become familiar with the applicable standard and see that it is implemented. Employees must be instructed regarding those safety standards that apply in their specific work areas.

The procedure for establishment of a standard is clearly defined in the legislation. Any plan by OSHA to develop, amend, or delete a standard must be announced in the *Federal Register.* A time period of at least 30 days must be given for public response and input. After this period of time a public hearing is scheduled by OSHA at which any interested party, individual, or organization, may request to present applicable data and information. Then within 60 days after the close of public hearings or the public comment period, OSHA will publish the new standard in the *Federal Register.* The full text of the standard will be published along with the date it is to become effective. Often the time lapse from the announcement of intent to establish a standard to the final publication of the standard may take months or even years.

Hazard Evaluations and Inspections

The Occupational Safety and Health Act authorizes the Occupational Safety and Health Administration (OSHA) to conduct hazard evaluations and to inspect workplaces. The purpose of such inspections is to ascertain the level of conformity to the various standards and to identify safety hazards. Any business or industry covered by the provisions of the legislation is subject to inspection.

Inspection Priorities Inspections are conducted by OSHA compliance officers who must undergo specific training to become familiar with all OSHA regulations. Because it is impossible to inspect all businesses and industries on a regular basis, OSHA has established a system of priorities for inspection. Top priority is given to those situations in which there is imminent danger to the life or physical well-being of the workers. These circumstances involve any conditions which might cause death or serious injury before the dangers can be eliminated.

The second priority is inspecting a workplace in which an accident has resulted in the death or the hospitalization of five or more employees. Whenever such an event takes place, OSHA must be informed within 48 hours. These inspections are directed toward determining if standards were violated, contributing to the catastrophe.

The third priority for OSHA inspections is directed toward employee complaints. Any worker has the right under provisions of this legislation to report a situation that seems to be in violation of standards. Importantly, no employer can penalize—either by dismissal or reduction in position or salary—an individual who has filed an unsafe standard complaint to OSHA. Many potentially dangerous situations have been identified through worker initiative.

OSHA has set another priority for inspection—that of high-risk industries, occupations, or working conditions. The selection of settings for inspection is established on the basis of likelihood of death, injury, and illness incidence rates.

A final emphasis is to conduct follow-up inspections. These are carried out to ascertain whether previously cited violations have been corrected. Failure to correct defects noted in a previous violation can result in additional penalties to the business or industry.

Inspection Procedures Since the legislation gives OSHA compliance officers the authority to monitor workplaces, the agency has set specific procedures for conducting such inspections. Most inspections are conducted without giving advance notice. Upon arrival at the company or industry, the compliance officer must show appropriate credentials. The officer then holds an opening conference with the appropriate company representative before beginning the inspection tour—informing the company representative of the purpose and scope of the inspection.

After this conference the compliance officer, accompanied by a company representative and a representative of the workforce, usually a labor representative, inspects the work site. The purpose of this tour is to ascertain the degree of compliance with OSHA standards. It is mandatory that any trade secrets observed by the compliance inspectors be kept confidential.

Upon completion of the inspection tour, a closing conference is held to discuss any related items that are pertinent to the inspection observations. At this time the compliance officer indicates violations that will be reported.

The OSHA compliance officer files a report on the inspection to the local area Occupational Safety and Health Administration office. The area director then has the authority to issue whatever citations seem appropriate and to level the related penalties. The penalty may be a monetary fine or a citation. Notification of each citation is sent to the employer, for posting at, or near, the work site where the deficiency was noted. In this way the workers are informed of the violation and of measures needed to correct the problem.

Labor or management can appeal the OSHA decision. Often an appeal can delay the corrective action or postpone payment of the fine.

Violations OSHA has established five classifications of violations. For each, specific monetary penalties have been determined. A *serious*

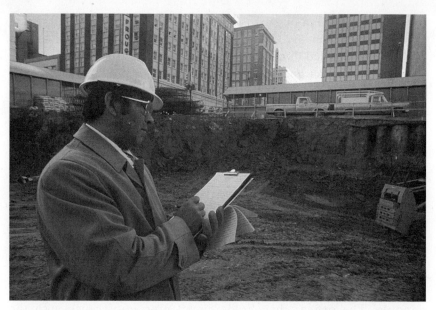
OSHA compliance officers conduct several different types of inspections in and around work sites.

violation means there is substantial probability that death or serious physical harm to employees could result and when the employer knew, or should have known, of the hazard. OSHA has identified a *willful violation* as a circumstance in which the employer intentionally and knowingly permits a hazardous condition to exist. In these situations the employer has made no reasonable effort to eliminate the hazard. Situations in which the compliance officer finds a violation similar to one previously cited are referred to as *repeat violations.* Another violation occurs when the employer *fails to correct prior violations.* The fifth classification of violations includes situations which are unacceptable under the law but which probably would not cause death or serious physical harm to the employees—known as *other than serious violations.*

Penalties   Maximum allowable penalties were increased significantly for all classifications of violations by Congress in 1991. Each willful or repeated violation now carries a maximum penalty of $70,000. Each other-than-serious violation now carries a maximum penalty of $7,000. The minimum penalty for a willful violation is now $5,000. An employer can be fined up to $7,000 for each instance of failure to post the OSHA report informing the employees of the violation and penalty.

Rights and Responsibilities

Under provisions of the Occupational Safety and Health Act both employers and employees have very clearly identified rights and responsibilities.

EMPLOYER RIGHTS AND RESPONSIBILITIES AS DEFINED UNDER OSHA

SELECTED RESPONSIBILITIES OF EMPLOYERS

The employer shall:
a. provide a hazard-free workplace.
b. be familiar and comply with mandatory OSHA standards.
c. make sure employees have and use safe equipment.
d. provide medical examinations required by OSHA standards.
e. keep proper records of work-related injuries.
f. post OSHA citations at, or near, the worksite involved.

SELECTED RIGHTS OF THE EMPLOYER

a. When an OSHA compliance officer comes, the employer has a right to know the reasons for the inspection and to have an opening and a closing conference.
b. Upon receipt of a notice of citation or penalty, the employer has the right to file a notice of contest.
c. The employer may apply for a permanent variance from a standard if proof can be furnished that the method of operation provides employee protection at least as effective as that required by the standard.
d. Confidentiality of all trade secrets observed by the compliance officer is guaranteed.

EMPLOYEE RIGHTS AND RESPONSIBILITIES AS DEFINED UNDER OSHA

SELECTED RESPONSIBILITIES OF EMPLOYEES

Employees shall:
a. comply with all OSHA standards.
b. read OSHA data as posted at the job site.
c. wear protective equipment while on the job.
d. report any job-related injury and seek treatment immediately.
e. cooperate with the OSHA compliance officer conducting an inspection.

SELECTED EMPLOYEE RIGHTS GUARANTEED BY THE ACT

a. Have protection against discharge, discrimination, or demotion because of filing a complaint against the employer.
b. May talk with the compliance officer and observe any monitoring or measuring action taken during an inspection.
c. Must be informed of any actions the employer plans to take resulting from an OSHA inspection.
d. May request information from an employer regarding hazards in the work area and precautions that may be taken.
e. Must receive information and training on workplace safety hazards.

Relationship of OSHA with the States

At the time of the passage of the Occupational Safety and Health Act there was much congressional opposition based upon the debate over federal government and state government control. Political compromise took place to gain the support of those members of Congress who wanted state control. It was agreed that individual states could develop and operate their own occupational safety and health programs.

Hence, states have the right to set their own standards and carry out enforcement measures separate from the federal Occupational Safety and Health Administration (OSHA). The federal government will provide up to 50 percent of the funding necessary for operation of the state-approved program. In order to receive OSHA approval a state program must be "as effective as" the federal government program. Administrative procedures must be adequate, enforcement measures must be identified, and standard-setting mechanisms must be effective. OSHA will continue to evaluate the individual state programs. If the state program is not deemed to be adequate, OSHA can reintroduce federal enforcement procedures.

In order to be approved, a state plan must show that within three years from the date of establishment, the plan can function as effectively as the federal program. States must provide appropriate legislation, guidelines, enforcement and appeals procedures, as well as related training, education, and technical assistance programs. When a state plan is approved, OSHA will limit its involvement to areas not covered in the state plan. All concurrent federal enforcement becomes the responsibility of the individual state. Whenever a state intends to change its plan, OSHA must be notified. There currently are 25 states with state plans. Twenty-three of these cover the private and public sectors, while two cover only the public sector.[13]

STATES WITH APPROVED OCCUPATIONAL SAFETY AND HEALTH PROGRAMS

Alaska	Maryland	South Carolina
Arizona	Michigan	Tennessee
California	Minnesota	Utah
Connecticut	Nevada	Vermont
Hawaii	New Mexico	Virginia
Indiana	New York	Washington
Iowa	North Carolina	Wyoming
Kentucky	Oregon	

Source: U.S. Department of Labor, Occupational Safety and Health Administration, *All About OSHA, 1991* (Revised).

Impact of OSHA

How effective has OSHA been? Has there been a reduction in the number of occupational fatalities and injuries since the implementation of the legislation in 1970? Can it be shown that work hours lost because of work-related injuries have been reduced? If so, is there evidence from research data proving that the reductions result from mandates in the legislation? Is the Occupational Safety and Health Administration another example of government bureaucracy establishing regulations that infringe upon the freedom of private business and industry? These are just a few examples of the many questions that have been discussed, debated, and argued relating to the effectiveness of OSHA.

Many differences of opinion can be found about the merits or drawbacks of OSHA. Some will emphasize that OSHA is nothing more than a federal agency designed to establish governmental control over business and industry. Those who hold to this view suggest that through the process of regulation, most small and medium-sized companies and industries are hurt. Independence is lost and cost inflation occurs as companies attempt to meet the demands of government. Such opponents of OSHA point out that employers are required to spend significant sums of money to produce only marginal safety benefits in the workplace.

OSHA regulations have had an impact upon business and industry, as well as the consumer, through the enforcement of costly changes in various manufacturing processes. Whenever safety measures are required to be instituted in the manufacturing process, the cost of implementing these procedures is usually passed on to the consumer in the price of the product.

There is some question whether any noticeable reduction in work-related fatalities and injuries has occurred since 1970. In 1970, some 14,000 workers were killed in job-related accidents; in addition, another 2.5 million workers were injured. The number of work-related fatalities in the early 1990s was about 8,500; however, the number of disabling injuries was more than three million.

Supporters of OSHA point to this kind of data as evidence of the effectiveness of safety programs designed under the mandate of legislation. Detractors suggest that in the years since World War II, long before the legislation, there had been a steady decrease in the death rates resulting from work-related accidents. In the mid-1940s death rates were 30 to 33 for every 100,000 workers. By the early 1990s the overall work-related death rate had dropped to nine per 100,000.[14]

Whether OSHA has been instrumental in reducing the numbers of work-related fatalities and injuries has not been answered conclusively. Certainly OSHA has contributed to a safer working place for many. Increased research has led to better understandings of dangerous conditions, substances, and environments in the occupational workplace. However, to "prove" that the statistical improvements are directly related to the legislation passed in 1970 is difficult, if not impossible.

Another controversial issue relating to the Occupational Safety and Health Act has centered on the inspection and enforcement procedures. Some people believe that OSHA inspectors are not knowledgeable in all aspects of the industrial safety field—hence, do not conduct adequate inspections.

Scattered among the thousands of individual standards that have been adopted are some whose merit and value must be questioned. Many are standards that have been in place for years but never have been enforced. For example, one outdated local standard prohibited placing ice in drinking water. This standard originated prior to the development of modern refrigerators and freezers when ice chopped from rivers was used to cool meats, dairy products, and drinks—a practice not considered to be sanitary.

Another criticism of OSHA has centered around the slowness of the standard setting process. For example, in the 1970s following several explosions involving grain storage facilities, OSHA conducted numerous grain elevator inspections and issued citations. At that time there were no established standards. Generally grain elevators explode because there are dangerous levels of airborne grain dust that ignite in the presence of an ignition source. The solution is to eliminate dust from the air and to control potential sources of ignition. It was not until 1987 that an OSHA standard was published that required the cleaning of surfaces of grain dust around grain storage facilities.

Critics of the penalty system point out that often when a penalty is imposed, the fine is so minimal as to result in little change of condition at the work site. Violation penalties also can be considered insignificant in view of the magnitude of the accident or the potential for injury or even death. OSHA administrators usually point out that the dollar value of fines are determined in relation to the severity of the violation; they never were intended to represent compensation for injury or loss of life to the individual and his or her family. In an attempt to stiffen the penalty system, Congress passed legislation in 1991 that increased the maximum limits for monetary penalties.

It is the feeling of many, including organized labor, that OSHA's effectiveness has been less than it should be, due in part to (1) weak enforcement procedures, (2) lack of skilled industrial safety and health personnel, and (3) the failure of the federal government to authorize an adequate budget to perform the needed tasks. This became particularly evident during the 1980s when workplace health and safety received a low federal governmental priority status. OSHA experienced significant budget and related staff cuts during these years. With reduced budget allocations it became difficult to carry out the many needed inspections and follow-up procedures that were considered to be important. As a result only the highest priorities of violations received attention.

OSHA reporting procedures also tend to cause disproportionate problems for small companies. Small businesses are affected more by injuries than larger companies and corporations, because they usually do not employ skilled personnel to investigate accidents. Lost work time usually results for management personnel when it is necessary to investigate the cause of an accident that in itself has resulted in lost work time. As a result, management of small businesses especially are under pressure to provide leadership in safety issues, to be alert to potential accidents, and provide training for all employees.

In spite of the many differences of opinion concerning the effectiveness of OSHA, it is important to recognize that the well-being and safety of all employees in business and industry must be the combined responsibility of management, labor, government, as well as each individual.

Occupational Safety Objectives for the Year 2000

Several of the occupational health and safety objectives for the year 2000 as published by the Public Health Service in 1990 relate to reducing fatalities and injuries at the work site. One objective calls for the reduction of fatalities from work-related injuries. In order to achieve the objective, four special worker population groups were identified as warranting specific initiatives during the 1990s. These target populations include employees engaged in mining, which has the highest ratio of fatalities per full-time worker, as well as construction workers, transportation workers, and agricultural employees.[15]

Other objectives addressed the need to reduce work-related injuries resulting in medical treatment and lost time from work. With as many as 10 million people suffering injuries on the job annually, the importance of this objective is understandable.[16]

Attention was also given to the need to reduce work-related cumulative trauma disorders.[17] These disorders result from repetitive motion that leads to pain, injury, and the inability to carry out one's work effectively. Two such disorders that result in significant amount of lost work time are back injuries and carpal tunnel syndrome.

The largest number of claims for workers' compensation—one-fourth of all claims—are for back injuries. The primary risk factor for back injuries is lifting. Stressful lifting results in mini-trauma to the tissues of the back. The effects of these mini-traumas accumulate with repetitive activity. Eventually, the basic anatomy of the back can become altered so that the range of motion is restricted. This can lead to long-term chronic back injury. Other common causes of such injuries include overextension, repeated activity, and exposure to vibrating machinery. Prolonged work postures, such as sitting at a computer or sorting mail in the post office for hours, are other risk factors associated with back trauma. Back injuries frequently are very painful and recovery can take a long period of time.

Another cumulative trauma disorder that has received considerable attention recently is carpal tunnel syndrome. This syndrome, one symptom of which is tingling in the fingers and hand, occurs because of excessive and continuous pressure on the median nerve at the point at which it passes through the narrow tunnel of bone and ligament of the wrist. This nerve supplies feeling to the hand; when it becomes compressed at the wrist, pain or numbness and weakness in the hand and thumb occur. Over a period of time if left untreated, carpal tunnel syndrome can lead to permanent dysfunction in the hand.

Individuals who are most commonly afflicted with carpal tunnel syndrome are persons whose work responsibilities involve repetitive wrist and hand motions. The condition is aggravated by vibration and tension from operating high-force machinery. It also occurs among clerical workers whose wrists are maintained in flexed positions for extensive periods of time. Carpal tunnel syndrome is treatable when diagnosis is made at an early stage. For cases of advanced syndrome, surgery and intensive rehabilitation may be helpful. However, preventive measures are important to protect against the possible development of chronic carpal tunnel syndrome and possible long-term disability.

Another of the national health objectives for the year 2000 addressed reduction of occupational skin disorders.[18] Each day many workers come into contact with chemicals, various materials, equipment, and conditions that can injure the skin. These skin injuries result in extensive amounts of lost work time and often the need for expensive medical care.

Minimizing skin disorders and related injuries in the workplace can best be achieved by requiring and providing protective clothing and by educating the employees about protecting the skin from chemical, physical, and mechanical agents. Every employer should not only take measures to provide a safe working environment, but should also inform the employees of potentially dangerous situations.

Personnel Involved in Occupational Safety

There are several professions that perform important roles in occupational safety. The most common are industrial hygienists, safety engineers, and occupational physicians and nurses.

Industrial Hygienists

The industrial hygienist is employed by many companies for the purpose of carrying out activities dealing with environmental factors at the work site that may cause injury or illness to the employees. Industrial hygienists usually have education, training, and experience that will enable them to carry out surveys and to analyze various potentially hazardous agents that can have a detrimental impact on the employees. Chemical, physical, toxic, and biological agents are of concern to the industrial hygienist. Not only are hygienists qualified to assess these hazardous agents, but they also have the responsibility of introducing and implementing programs that are designed to control these workplace hazards.

The industrial hygienist must be familiar with the many federal exposure limits that have been established for chemicals, toxic substances, and biological agents. Where these substances exceed the federally mandated exposure limits, the industrial hygienist must recommend measures to remove the hazard or to substitute a less hazardous material into the manufacturing process.

Safety Engineers

The safety engineer is trained to identify potential hazards in the workplace that can cause injury to the working man or woman. Once the potentially hazardous conditions are identified, the safety engineer must recommend measures that can be taken to eliminate or neutralize them.

In many corporate settings the safety engineer has the responsibility for developing safety education programs for employees. These programs usually emphasize accident prevention and the development and maintenance of a safe working environment.

Occupational Physicians and Nurses

Medical doctors or registered nurses who are trained as specialists in occupational illnesses and injuries are known as occupational physicians and occupational nurses. Such a physician usually serves as the medical director for the health program of the company or industry of which he or she is employed. The occupational nurse carries out a variety of primary health care activities for employees at the workplace.

Both occupational physicians and occupational nurses must be familiar with the specific harmful substances and working conditions in the place of employment. In addition to providing primary health care to employees, they also work to reduce potential job site hazards. Educational initiatives for employees about various workplace hazards are often organized and carried out by such occupational medical personnel.

An important benefit of the Occupational Safety and Health Act has been the establishment of educational training programs for all industrial health and safety personnel. For example, workshops, in-service training programs, and academic courses of study have been developed to educate more effective safety and health personnel for the workplace. Degree programs also have been established at both the undergraduate and graduate levels in such areas of study as industrial hygiene, occupational nursing, and safety engineering. In order to secure employment, occupational health and safety personnel must be properly certified and licensed.

Selected Work Sites

It is not possible within the framework of this chapter to consider the dimensions of safety and accident prevention for all occupational settings. Two occupational settings in which fatality and injury are all too common have been selected for discussion. Obviously different degrees of danger exist in the varied areas of work where one might be employed. It is the responsibility of all persons to become familiar with regulations and standards that apply to their workplaces. In turn, practicing those measures can go a long way in improving the safety records of the workplace.

Mining

Possibly the most dangerous American industry from the viewpoint of work-related injury and fatalities is mining—a field employing approximately 400,000 workers in the United States. The nature of mining and the hostile environment in which workers must spend most of each working day contribute to the high fatality and injury rates. According to the National Safety Council, the mining industry has the highest death rate next to agriculture—29 deaths per 100,000 miners—of all industries.[19]

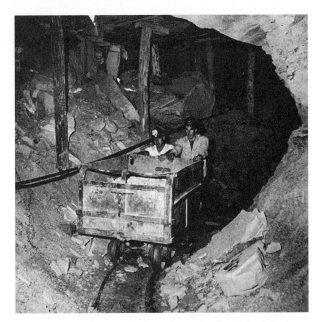

Mining has the highest death rate of any industry in the United States.

Safety records are much better for surface than for underground mining operations. Coal mining is the most hazardous of all underground mining operations. Coal mining permits little room for error. Seldom does a year pass without a coal mining accident that results in multiple fatalities.

Coal miners often must work in wet, damp, constrained working environments. Included in the coal mining environment is the use of various tools, such as pneumatic drills, hammers, automated screw drivers, scaling bars, and other high-speed equipment that can cause serious injury. Work in a mine usually takes place with limited illumination. In coal mines the battery-powered light on the hard hat provides the only light for many employees.

In an underground mining environment, fires and explosions cause the greatest number of fatalities; most often injuries in coal mining are the result of falling debris from the roof of the mine, transportation accidents within the mine, and machinery- and electrical-related accidents. Danger is also associated with the unstable underground rocks that may fall upon workers. Other types of injuries occur from the lifting, pulling, and pushing of material. Slips and falls also cause a variety of work-related injuries.

Safety in the Workplace—Economic as Well as Personal Concerns

Fires and explosions result from the release of explosive gas. In coal mining the danger of methane gas, emitted from a coal seam as mining takes place, is of great concern. As long as there is good ventilation in the mine, the liberated gas is diluted to a level below the explosion point. However, without proper ventilation, dilution does not occur and a tragic explosion may result. Research and development are providing new, improved means of ventilation in many mines.

In mine accidents, lives are frequently lost and serious injuries sustained because there is no rapid emergency rescue procedure. It is important that trapped miners be located as rapidly as possible. A system of seismic locators has been developed to help locate trapped miners. Another rescue measure is the development of a "probe hole," a small hole drilled to the location of the trapped miners, through which food and other supplies can be lowered. It is also possible to lower a closed-circuit television camera and ascertain the condition of the mine to determine further rescue efforts that can be taken.

The mining industry is regulated by standards authorized by the Federal Coal Mine Health and Safety Act which established a national code for the coal mine industry. The Mining Enforcement Safety and Health Administration was initially created from mandates of this legislation. Today, this federal administrative agency is known as the Mine Safety and Health Administration. It is a part of the Department of Labor.

The Mine Safety and Health Administration has authority to inspect mines and to close all or any part of a mine that is considered to be dangerous. This agency has authority to enforce all safety policies. For example, tunnels in mines must be covered with rock dust made from ground limestone. This protects against the spread of fire should an explosion occur. Another policy states that company inspectors must examine the working areas three hours before each shift to ensure mine safety.

In considering problems related to mine safety, one cannot overlook the importance of safety instruction and continuing education programs for all those who work in mines. Training and educating new miners is particularly important as new mine employees are much more likely to experience an injury-producing situation than are experienced miners. New miners must have at least 40 hours of training in self-rescue, first aid, and other safety measures. Also periodic refresher courses in safety are now mandated for most mine employees.[20]

Transportation

According to data from the Department of Transportation, more than 1,200 drivers of trucks are fatally injured each year. These involve operators of medium and tractor-trailer trucks. Many other individuals are killed and injured resulting from collisions with trucks.

There are federal and state laws designed to improve the safety record of the trucking industry. For example, commercial drivers are expected to make a safety check before each trip. Brakes, steering, lights, tires, reflectors, horns, wipers, coupling devices, and fire extinguishers should all be checked. Federal regulations require that drivers of trucks weighing 10,000 or more pounds cannot drive more than ten hours without an eight hour rest period. They also are not supposed to drive more than 60 hours within seven consecutive days. Truckers are prohibited from drinking alcohol within four hours of entering their cab. This is one of the provisions of the Commercial Driver's License Act, administered by the various states, but mandated by the federal government.[21] All commercial truck drivers must pass a written knowledge test and a road skill test. Standards for this examination have been issued by the Federal Highway Administration.

Deregulation of the trucking industry during the 1980s resulted in the establishment of smaller trucking companies and the growth of the independent trucker. The outcome has been increased numbers of inexperienced drivers on the highways. Many trucking companies have been known to cut safety corners; some cannot afford the costs of safety training and other important prevention measures.

Employee Occupational Safety Initiatives

Many different activities, programs, and approaches are used to encourage safety in the industrial and occupational setting. Safety posters and slogans draw the attention of the employee. Planned training initiatives in proper equipment operational procedures are helpful in promoting safety in the workplace. However, safety instruction and training in the occupational setting involve more than imparting facts or information about how to perform a certain procedure. They focus on the positive—emphasizing why an action is important. Workers must be motivated to put safety training into practice.

Personal Protective Equipment

An important measure designed to protect the working individual in most industrial settings is the requirement that certain personal protective pieces of equipment must be worn. Such equipment includes wearing gloves, safety shoes, jackets, protective eye glasses, ear plugs, and hard hats.

The wearing of hard hats on the job is not a twentieth-century development. As early as 1586 Italians working on St. Peter's Cathedral in Rome were ordered to wear battle helmets to protect their heads from injury.[22] However, since the passage of the Occupational Safety and Health Act, a greater number of industrial workers are protected by the mandated use of the hard hat. These hats must be comfortable as well as strong enough to protect the wearer from injury due to falling objects in the work environment.

People tend to resist change that conflicts with their normal behavioral patterns. For this reason, it has not always been easy to get employees to want to use personal protective equipment, and many objections have been raised regarding mandatory use of the equipment. For example, those who oppose the use of hard hats say that they are uncomfortable or hot; others say that they interfere with their working ability.

Efforts designed to gain acceptance of personal protective equipment by employees include a number of different measures. Organized labor has been very supportive in these efforts. Employer recognition of positive safety behavior by workers is also helpful.

Not only does industry have a responsibility to provide required protective equipment, but it has an obligation to make certain that such equipment is used. An employer cannot assume that once the employee has the equipment, the company's responsibility ends. Industry must make sure that the equipment is used and worn properly.

Employee Motivational Programs

Many companies have established incentive programs to supplement their ongoing safety initiatives. These programs vary widely. Some emphasize activities that motivate employees to become more safety conscious. Others are more recognition-oriented; employees are rewarded for actions they have taken that contribute to safety in their workplace.

An effective employee safety motivational program must be attractive to the employee.[23] The workers must be made to feel that they share responsibility for carrying out the particular initiatives.

The particular reward system used also must have meaning to the workers involved in the program. For instance, money is often the reward that is made available. Such an incentive has its drawbacks, however. Employees may wish to obtain the monetary reward, but all too often this will not create an internal desire to achieve a safe environment that prevails when the reward is not available. Recognition by management and one's superiors, as well as colleagues, is often the best type of award in an employee motivation program. When personal behavior is reinforced at this level, ongoing safety consciousness is most likely to result.[24]

Summary

Accurate data on the total number of fatalities and injuries occurring in occupational settings is hard to obtain. What is known is that many workers are involved in on-the-job accidents each working day. The results are fatality, injury, and economic losses.

Historically, there have been numerous initiatives designed to provide a safer workplace. In 1970 the United States Congress passed the Occupational Safety and Health Act. This legislation was designed to reduce injuries and fatalities in the workplace. Two federal agencies were created out of the mandate of this act: the Occupational Safety and Health Administration (OSHA) and the National Institute of Occupational Safety and Health (NIOSH).

Guidelines have been established for inspection priorities and for the conduct of such inspections by OSHA compliance officers. Under provisions of the legislation, both the employee and the employer have clearly defined rights and responsibilities.

The federal government has established several health objectives to be achieved by the year 2000 relating to safety in the workplace. These objectives are to reduce fatalities from work-related injuries, to reduce work-related injuries necessitating medical treatment, and to decrease lost time from work. Also attention is aimed at reducing cumulative trauma disorders—particularly back injuries and carpal tunnel syndrome.

In order to minimize personal injury and fatality, employees must use personal protective equipment and should be educated and involved through ongoing safety motivation initiatives. Measures must be identified to encourage the use of hard hats, protective gloves, safety boots, and eyeglasses.

Only as individuals come to accept the need for safe practices in the workplace will the number of fatalities and injuries occurring at work be reduced. Continued efforts from management, labor, the individual employee, as well as government mandates are necessary.

Discussion Questions

1. What is the extent of workplace fatalities and injuries in the United States? Support your answer with statistical data.
2. Trace some of the historical development of occupational safety initiatives during the 1800s and in the early 1900s.
3. What is worker's compensation insurance?
4. What was significant about the First Cooperative Safety Congress held in 1912?
5. Discuss some of the factors that developed from the passage of the Occupational Safety and Health Act of 1970.
6. Explain how safety standards are established by the Occupational Safety and Health Administration (OSHA).
7. What priorities has OSHA established for conducting workplace inspections?
8. Discuss the five different classifications of violations of workplace safety.
9. What are the responsibilities of an OSHA compliance officer?
10. Why was provision made in the Occupational Safety and Health Act for states to establish state OSHA agencies?
11. Do you believe that the Occupational Safety and Health Act has been a useful mechanism for improving occupational safety or not? Defend your answer.
12. Discuss the national health and safety objectives for the year 2000 that apply to occupational safety.
13. What is carpal tunnel syndrome?
14. What measures should be taken to provide for a safer mining work environment?
15. What measures can be taken to encourage workers to use personal protective equipment?

Suggested Readings

Bjornstig, Ulf, and Jeanette Johnsson. "Ladder Injuries: Mechanisms, Injuries, and Consequences," *Journal of Safety Research* 23, no. 1 (Spring 1992): 9–18.

Campany, Sarah O., and Martin E. Personick. "Profiles in Safety and Health: Retail Grocery Sales," *Monthly Labor Review* 115, no. 9 (September 1992): 9–16.

Castelli, Jim. "What the Future Holds for OSHA," *Safety and Health* 147, no. 1 (January 1993): 40–43.

Castelli, Jim. "What's the State of State OSHA Plans," *Safety and Health* 145, no. 6 (June 1992): 66–69.

Daltroy, Lawren H. "Teaching and Social Support: Effects on Knowledge, Attitudes, and Behaviors to Prevent Low Back Injuries in Industry," *Health Education Quarterly* 20, no. 1 (Spring 1993): 43–62.

Geddes, Annmarie L. "Below the Surface," *Ohio Monitor* 64, no. 5 (May 1991): 16–21.

Hawkins, Jeff. "Safe and Healthy Workers Deserve Recognition," *Safety and Health* 138, no. 1 (July 1988): 34–36.

Kraus, Jess F. "Homicide While at Work: Persons, Industries, and Occupations at High Risk," *American Journal of Public Health* 77, no. 10 (October 1987): 1285–89.

Lahey, James W. "Hands: the $5.5 Billion Challenge," *Safety and Health* 137, no. 6 (June 1988): 36–38.

Melia, Marilyn Kennedy. "Occupational Health Nurses: Good Medicine for the Workplace," *Safety and Health* 149, no. 5 (May 1994): 76–79.

Personick, Martin E., and Laura A. Harthun. "Profiles in Safety and Health: the Soft Drink Industry," *Monthly Labor Review* 115, no. 4 (April 1992): 12–17.

Shi, Leiyu. "A Cost-Benefit Analysis of a California County's Back Injury Program," *Public Health Reports* 108, no. 2 (March–April, 1993): 204–11.

Slappendel, Carol, and others. "Factors Affecting Work-Related Injury Among Forestry Workers: A Review," *Journal of Safety Research* 24, no. 1 (Spring 1993): 19–32.

Toscano, Guy, and Janice Windau. "Fatal Work Injuries: Census for 31 States," *Monthly Labor Review* 115, no. 9 (September 1992): 3–8.

Tyson, Patrick R. "OSHA Reform: The Stage Is Set for the Showdown," *Safety and Health* 149, no. 5 (May 1994): 31–34.

Wolnez, George J. "Challenge the Conventional Wisdom on Back Injuries," *Safety and Health* 149, no. 5 (May 1994): 92–93.

Endnotes

1. Department of Health and Human Services, *Healthy People 2000: National Health Promotion and Disease Prevention Objectives* (Washington DC: U.S. Government Printing Office, 1991), 296.
2. Guy Toscano and Janice Windau, "Fatal Work Injuries: Census for 31 States," *Monthly Labor Review* 115, no. 9 (September 1992): 3–8.
3. Ibid.
4. National Safety Council, *Accident Facts, 1993 Edition* (Itasca, IL: National Safety Council, 1993), 34.
5. Ibid., 111.
6. Ibid., 35.
7. Ibid.
8. "America's Accomplishments in Safety—The First 200 Years," *Professional Safety* 21, no. 4 (April 1976): 19.
9. Ibid., 19.
10. Ibid., 20–21.
11. The term *worker's compensation* replaces the older term "workmen's compensation" to reflect the presence of females in the workplace.
12. National Safety Council, *Accident Facts 1993*, 43.
13. Department of Labor, *All About OSHA, 1991, rev.* (Washington, DC: U.S. Government Printing Office, 1991).
14. National Safety Council, *Accident Facts 1993*, 34.
15. Department of Health and Human Services, *Healthy People 2000: National Health Promotion and Disease Prevention Objectives,* (Washington, DC: U.S. Government Printing Office, 1991): 298.
16. Ibid., 299.
17. Ibid., 300.

18. Ibid., 300–301.
19. National Safety Council, *Accident Facts 1993,* 34.
20. Annmarie L. Geddes, "Below the Surface," *Ohio Monitor* 64, no. 5 (May 1991): 16–21.
21. Contact your local Division of Motor Vehicles or Secretary of State for additional information about the Commercial Driver's License.
22. Nancy L. Nelson, "Safety Starts at the Top," *Job Safety and Health* 1, no. 1 (November–December 1972): 3.
23. Jeff Hawkins, "Safe and Healthy Workers Deserve Recognition," *Safety and Health* 138, no. 1 (July 1988): 34–36.
24. Ibid.

CHAPTER 6

Rural Safety—Working and Living in the Rural Environment

Chapter Outline

Introduction
Injury in the Rural Setting
Government Regulation and Agriculture
Farm Machinery
   Risk Factors Associated with Farm Machinery
   Power-Driven Machine Components
   Tractors
Grain Storage
   Fire
   Entrapment
   Lack of Ventilation
Exposure to Toxic Gases
Danger of Chemicals
Electrocution and Electrical Shock
Safety Concerns in Other Rural Occupations
Summary
Discussion Questions
Suggested Readings
Endnotes

Introduction

The rural setting seems to many to be a place of tranquility, quiet, peace, and protection from many of the stresses related to urban living. In recent years many urban dwellers have moved from the major metropolitan areas of the country to small communities. Many have settled on acreage where they have taken up an agricultural life-style.

To the person unfamiliar with problems related to rural living, it may appear that there is little danger of injury and disability in such ostensibly idealic settings. Yet agricultural activities are among the most dangerous of occupations.[1] It is estimated that 1,300 fatalities occur among agriculture workers annually. Deaths among farm residents on an annual basis occur at the rate of 37 per 100,000 population, exceeding the construction industry's mortality rate of 32 and mining's rate of 29.[2] Compared with other industries such as the trade and manufacturing occupations (with fatality rates of 4 and 3 respectively), agriculture is statistically a very dangerous occupation.

Not only is the death rate high among agricultural workers, but the incidence of disabling injuries is a serious problem as well. More than 270,000 farm residents sustained disabling work-related injuries in one recent year.

A disabling injury presents serious problems for the wage earner in any vocation. However, it is of particular difficulty for the agricultural worker. Farming is a self-contained business for many rural residents. Personal physical disability can mean a serious economic setback. Many times the rancher or farmer does not have adequate insurance to provide an income if he or she becomes disabled. Following an injury it is necessary for the work to be carried out by family and friends. For most farm workers the peak employment season spans a limited period of time. Should one become disabled during planting and harvesting, livelihood for the entire year may be jeopardized.

Injury in the Rural Setting

Many reasons can be given for the high incidence of fatalities and injuries among rural residents, particularly among agricultural employees. American agriculture in the 1990s, unlike years ago, is highly mechanized. Large combines, different sizes and kinds of tractors, cornpickers, hay balers, and various other types of mechanized equipment have been invented since the manufacture of the first reaper by Cyrus McCormick in the last century. Improved mechanization of farm equipment, though of inestimable value to the farmer's economic productivity, is a major contributor to incidents which result in fatality, injury, and disability.

Farmers often work alone, particularly when out in their fields. When a circumstance arises that causes injury, often a lengthy period of time can pass until help arrives. Such delay in obtaining necessary aid and medical assistance often seriously compounds the physical problems involved in the situation.

Weather is another factor contributing to unsafe agricultural work conditions. It is not unusual for a farmer to get behind in planting or harvesting due to inclement weather. Under the stress of these conditions an individual is likely to take chances and an injury producing situation may result. Fatigue and reduced judgment combine to worsen already dangerous working conditions.

In most occupational settings today safety programs have been designed to inform and educate employees who are exposed to highly mechanized equipment, dangerous substances, and other hazards to which individuals are exposed at the work site. This has not always been the case in agriculture. Farming traditionally has been an independent operation, and supervision, training, and the enforcement of laws and regulations have not always been effective. There is no supervisor present to ensure that preventive safety practices are followed. For example, it is nearly impossible to make sure that the farmer using a tractor is wearing a safety belt or that the cornpicker has the proper mechanized safeguards in place at all times. Though the operator of a mechanized piece of equipment has read the manufacturer's operating instructions, there is no guarantee that the recommended safety procedures will be followed once the farmer is working alone in the field.

Farmers and ranchers often resent rules and regulations imposed by governmental agencies—whether federal, state, or local—as an intrusion into their personal lifestyle. Economically they will point out that, unlike other businesses and industries, they cannot pass on the costs of added safety equipment and items mandated by governmental regulatory agencies to the consumer. Unfortunately, the agricultural worker does not consider the long-term potential costs associated with injury and disability; the focus centers basically only on those immediate out-of-pocket expenses related to meeting regulations and mandates.

On many family owned and operated farms young people help with the farming activities. Often these individuals lack experience and training to operate the machinery in a safe manner. Injury also occurs when young people come into contact with livestock. Feeding and handling of animals, particularly cows and horses, can result in serious injury if the individual does not take adequate care.

It is not unusual to see young people, sometimes as young as elementary school age, helping with the farming activities. Children between the ages of 5 and 14 have the highest farm injury rate of any other age group. There is no law that prohibits children from working on their own family farm. Also, by federal law, young people 12 years of age or older can work on other farms with a parent's permission. In short, it is difficult to stop the tradition of children performing farming chores. Many would argue that this is a good experience—a way of developing an important "work ethic."

Given such a prevailing mind-set, the need for effective farm safety education programs for young people is of major importance. In most rural communities the Future Farmers of America (FFA) and/or the 4-H Clubs provide effective safety education initiatives.

Many injuries occur to individuals who are part-time or weekend farmers who own some acreage in the country. During the day, these individuals work full-time in industry, commerce, or the professions, usually in the city. After a full day's employment, they go to their fields and put in many additional long hours during the evenings and on weekends. Here, too, fatigue can lead to incidents resulting in fatality and injury.

It is not unusual for these part-time farmers to have equipment that is old, used, and in need of repair. Such individuals usually have minimal experience in operation and maintenance of that equipment. All too often when the machinery breaks down, the individual attempts to repair it with little knowledge and skill as to the appropriate safety measures. Injuries to various parts of the body can occur, with the legs, head, fingers, and feet most commonly affected.

Government Regulation and Agriculture

Historically, agriculture has been virtually nonregulated in the area of safety. Research about safety in the agricultural workplace has not been a high priority—an important factor explaining why there is less government regulation in agriculture than in other occupational settings. For example, no federal governmental agency is charged officially with conducting agricultural safety research. Commonly, fatality and injury prevention initiatives have been carried out by state and local government farm organizations and voluntary farm organizations.

The Occupational Safety and Health Administration (OSHA) has published several regulations relating to agriculture, all designed to improve the safety of the farm employee. However, a number of problems impede attempts to improve the accident record among farmworkers. As an example, in 1976 OSHA issued regulations that all manufacturers of farm tractors must install rollover bars and provide seat belts on their products. However, until a 1984 law prohibited it, farmers could have these bars removed when purchasing a new vehicle. Now at least they cannot be removed upon purchase, but what happens once the piece of equipment is out in the field still is not mandated.

One of the major problems with the OSHA regulations relating to agricultural workers is that individuals working on farms with 10 or fewer employees are exempted from OSHA regulations. The majority of agricultural workers, as many as 90 percent, are to be found on small, family farms—hence, are exempt from these regulations. If a farmer does all the work on a farm or ranch without the help of others, except for family members, the regulations also do not apply.

Two OSHA standards that are significant for agricultural settings are the Field Sanitation Standard and the Hazard Communication Standard. The Field Sanitation Standard requires farmers employing field laborers to provide potable drinking water, toilets, and hand washing facilities at the work site. However, this standard applies to hand laborers in the fields, not to machine operators.

The Hazard Communication Standard applies to situations where workers are exposed to hazardous materials. Safety data sheets must be provided, containers must be labeled, and employees must be instructed about dangers and safety procedures when handling herbicides, insecticides, rodenticides, solvents, and fuels.

Even though many farm employees are not mandated to be covered by the OSHA regulations, it is important nonetheless that the guidelines be implemented by everyone. This is particularly true with regulations concerning safety guards and shields on movable parts of power machinery.

Unfortunately, a number of the rules and regulations established by OSHA have met with firm opposition by the farmers and ranchers—especially those which might seem to place controls and standards over their operational activities. Farm employers traditionally view such efforts by OSHA as an invasion of privacy. They resent anything that appears to be outside meddling, particularly when the activities, rules, and regulations are developed by bureaucratic officials with little or no farming experience.

Farm Machinery

Without modern high-speed machines, farming and ranching would not be the business it is today. Such equipment makes it possible for an individual to farm hundreds, even thousands of acres in an efficient and economic manner.

Risk Factors Associated with Farm Machinery

High-speed machines used in agriculture cause many injuries each year. A typical problem occurs when the operator tries to remove something that is clogged in the rotating machinery. Other hazardous situations involve attempts to repair an engine while it is still running. Any piece of farm machinery should be stopped whenever it is necessary to repair or adjust the equipment. This is true also whenever measures must be taken to unclog something that has become stuck. Failure to take measures to protect against injury from mechanized farm machinery represents carelessness on the part of the operator; the individual is in a hurry and simply fails to shut down the machine.

Over the winter months most farm equipment sits idle. It is important that measures be taken prior to the spring planting season to make sure that all engines and movable parts are serviced and maintained. Properly functioning machinery helps to protect against accidents. For example, cutting blades should be sharpened, which enables crops to be cut cleanly and reduces clogging.

Power-Driven Machine Components

To protect against injuries from farm machinery, OSHA regulations require that guards be placed on all power transmission and functioning components of farm equipment. Power takeoff (PTO) shafts and rotating drive lines must be covered by protective shields. The power takeoff shaft which channels power from the tractor to attached implements revolves at a very high rate of speed, from 9 to 17 revolutions per second. The revolving shaft can catch things—such as lines, ropes, loose clothing, and almost any other item that a person may be wearing—and in a matter of seconds can wrap a trapped person around the shaft. Protective shielding on this type of machinery should never be removed.

Any farmer who hires help must fit all farm equipment with injury-preventing safety shields. Shields are mandatory at the mesh points of power-driven chains, gears, belts, and pulleys. It is the employer's responsibility to make certain that the guards are in place and that all employees are informed of the safety features. The farmer also must instruct employees on how to use and service the power equipment.

Any machinery that has parts which continue to move after the power is shut off must be equipped with a warning device, either a visible or an audible signal. Work on the machinery should wait until the moving parts are no longer operating; measures also need to be taken to assure that the machine will not be started while repairs are being made.

Electrically powered equipment must be equipped with a disconnect device that prevents the machine from starting up accidentally when a worker is repairing, unclogging, adjusting, or servicing the

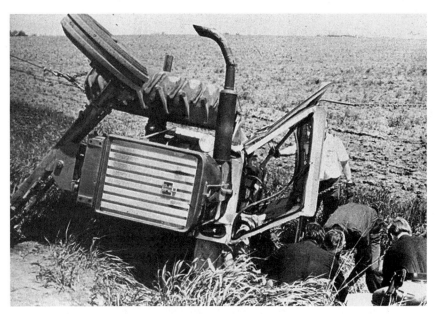

A leading cause of injury and death in rural localities results from tractors overturning.

machine. To prevent a motor from resetting and starting while a person is working on the machine, it is necessary to have a manual reset circuit.

Far too many fatalities and injuries occur to children and young people playing and working around farm machinery. It is particularly important to keep all young children off such equipment, even when it is not in operation.

Tractors

Of all the machinery used in agriculture, the tractor is the most common. It is operated more hours a day than is any other type of farm machinery. Tractors come in many different sizes and styles. There are large, cabin-style tractors that have a great amount of power. Other tractors are rather small in nature, such as those used in orchards, green houses, and in indoor warehouse and storage facilities. Because they are used more widely than any other types of equipment, more fatalities and injuries result from tractor use than from any other kind of farm machinery. The National Safety Council estimates that slightly more than 300 tractor-related fatalities occur annually.[3] Three major causes of tractor-related fatalities and injuries are *tractor overturns, falls from tractors,* and *on-road accidents.*

Rural Safety—Working and Living in the Rural Environment

Overturns

As many as half of all tractor-related fatalities result from overturns. There are two types of overturns: the side overturn and the rear overturn. Most tractor overturns occur on inclines in the terrain of the land. The side overturn occurs when the tractor is driven too close to sloped ditches, when crossing a slope, or when making a sharp turnaround. It is particularly dangerous to drive a tractor laterally on a slope that is greater than 25 percent. Tractors tend to be sensitive to shifts in their balance points. A shift occurs when the center of gravity moves beyond the plane containing the imaginary line connecting the outer edge of each wheel and running along the axles.[4]

The tractor is likely to go into a rear overturn when going up a slope, when the rear wheels become mired in mud, or when the hitch of a wagon or other piece of machinery or farm implement being pulled is positioned at a point too high on the rear of the tractor. Fast acceleration also may lead to a rear overturn.

A variety of situations can cause a tractor to turn over. When stuck in mud, the operator often opens the throttle full force in an effort to become unstuck. If the wheels remain mired when the power is applied, the chassis revolves around the axle and flips the tractor over backward. The same situation may occur when climbing up a steep embankment or pulling a heavy load with a high drawbar. Whenever it is necessary to pull heavy loads, the hitch should be kept low and front-end weights should be used. Any high-speed operation of the tractor over rough terrain may result in a turnover.

Any person operating a tractor should take measures to avoid a turnover. Such precautions include not operating the tractor near holes or depressions in the ground, on embankments, or near ditches. When it is necessary to use the tractor on a slope, it is important to know whether it is safe to operate on the existing slope. The operator should always reduce tractor speeds when driving on wet or muddy surfaces.

It is particularly important to be aware of speed when making a turn with a tractor. Turning too rapidly can result in a turnover. Operators of all tractors must learn the turning characteristics of each specific tractor they are driving.

Some people are of the opinion that should they become involved in an overturn situation they will be able to jump to safety before the tractor falls on them. This is very unlikely. It is estimated that most overturns occur in one to three seconds.[5] This obviously means that the tractor has turned over on the driver before he or she has time to react. Also, if it were possible that a person could jump from a tractor as it turned over, the likelihood of being run over by an implement being pulled is very high.

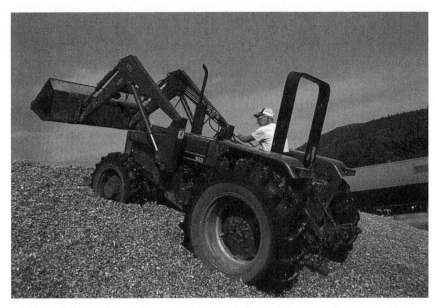

The rollover protection structure (ROPS) provides protection to the tractor operator should the tractor roll over.

Rollover Protective Structures (ROPS) In order to reduce injuries and fatalities resulting from tractor overturns, regulations have been established that require tractors to have rollover protective structures (ROPS) built into the frame of the vehicle. These structures are metal frame bars that limit the roll of the tractor to 90 degrees, preventing the tractor from turning upside down and crushing the driver. In addition to providing protection against a complete overturn, the ROPS tends to create greater tractor stability. This is because the center of gravity is shifted due to the increased height of the structure. It also adds to the weight of the tractor, further improving stability. With greater tractor stability the possibility of a tractor turning over is lessened.

The simplest type of tractor ROPS is the two-post system consisting of two steel posts mounted vertically over the rear axle of the tractor, with a steel beam mounted horizontally as a connector between the two posts. The four-post ROPS system has two additional vertical posts mounted near the front axle. This creates a cube structure which can be enclosed as a cab in which the operator sits.

There has been increasing use of larger all-purpose tractors with heated and air-conditioned cabs. These kinds of structures make it easier to build in the ROPS safety system.

Opposition to the ROPS system has centered on the fact that the installation results in a taller structure. This problem is particularly of concern to workers around greenhouses, or in orchards and vineyards. The added height of the structure can cause fruit to be knocked off low hanging limbs or tree limbs to be damaged. Similar concern has been expressed where tractors are used in and around buildings with low garage doorways. In order to help solve these problems, adjustable ROPS systems have been developed for use with small utility tractors. With these systems the structure can be telescoped or folded into a lower position, reducing the overall height.

OSHA standards require that all employees be instructed in ways to avoid a tractor turnover. Today all new tractors of more than 20 horsepower must have ROPS equipment as well as seat belts when used by an employee on a farm.

Seat Belts Not only is the ROPS system a vital safety feature on tractors, but the use of seat belts is also important. It is now mandatory that seat belts be installed and worn on tractors. However, many agricultural workers still do not use them. The opposition to their use is based on the idea that an operator is in and out of the cab or off the tractor seat so often that seat belts are viewed as being a bother. In efforts designed to encourage the increased use of seat belts, many rural safety proponents are including instruction about the need for seat belt use in classes for agricultural workers and for rural young people.

Falls from Tractors

Often fatalities and injuries occur when a person riding on the tractor falls and is either run over by the wheels or is injured falling to the ground. Though these situations occur to all age groups, all too frequently young children are involved.

The best way to protect against such occurrences is to never allow a second person to ride on the tractor. Tractors do not have seats to safely transport persons other than the vehicle operator. Danger also exists in permitting persons to ride on wagons and other vehicles being pulled by the tractor.

Anyone operating a tractor must be alert to external objects that can knock a person to the ground. Limbs on a tree or overhead wires can cause serious injuries and fatalities. Whenever the tractor must navigate over rough surfaces, driving at a reduced rate of speed protects the operator from being thrown from the vehicle.

On-Road Accidents

Although most farm work takes place off the roads and highways, it is sometimes necessary to drive tractors and other farm equipment in traffic. Special care must be taken whenever one is driving slow-moving vehicles on public roadways. As with any kind of vehicular driving, all traffic laws, road signs, and regulations must be obeyed.

Every slow-moving piece of farm machinery must display a special emblem that makes it easy to notice the vehicle. Any vehicle that travels 25 miles per hour or less is considered to be a slow-moving vehicle and must display the appropriate emblem. This emblem must be kept clean and be visible at all times. Because most collisions between motor vehicles and slow-moving farm equipment on public roadways occur during daylight hours, the slow-moving vehicle warning emblem must be effective in daylight as well as at night. In addition, the operator should have flashing warning lights operating at all times when operating on a public roadway.

Children must not be permitted to drive farm vehicles on the open road. This becomes a problem when a teenager is helping, as often occurs with farm work. The individual should not drive on the road unless he or she has a driver's license or unless the individual has had proper instruction through such agencies as the Future Farmers of America (FFA) or the 4-H Club. Some states now require a tractor operator to have a license if the person is going to operate the vehicle anywhere other than on his or her own family property.

Grain Storage

Large amounts of grain are stored on farms in storage bins and in silos. Many small communities scattered throughout rural America have commercial grain storage facilities. Such grain storage may present a variety of hazards, leading to fires, entrapment, suffocation, injury, and death.

Fire

The possibility of destructive fire is one major problem associated with grain storage facilities. There are a number of possible causes of such fires. Many silo fires occur when the silage stored is overly dry. As it ferments over time, low-moisture silage becomes hot. Fire results when such silage is mixed with oxygen from air leaks. Silo fires may smolder for extended periods of time before erupting into a major, destructive fire.

Fire may also occur as the result of an explosion when grain moving through the pipes in a storage bin create static electricity. Dust explosions may occur whenever grain dust, oxygen, and some source of energy are present. According to the National Fire Prevention

Association, such explosions occur in a chain reaction. The initial occurrence is rather small—perhaps jarring dust particles from ledges and beams in the storage bin or silo. This action, in turn, creates a cloud of dust, resulting in a more serious explosion. The spark from static electricity combined with the grain dust present in the air can very easily cause an explosion more powerful than dynamite.

The best protection against such explosions is keeping the grain storage bin well ventilated and clean. Grain dust should be removed whenever accumulation exceeds one-eighth inch. Electrical wiring must be maintained properly, and smoking must be prohibited in the storage area. Reducing the likelihood of destructive explosions can be enhanced by enclosing conveyor systems. Extreme care must be taken whenever mechanical, electrical, hydraulic, or pneumatic equipment is used inside storage bins or silos.

Entrapment

Personnel working in and around grain storage facilities must exercise caution because of the hazards of entrapment under tons of flowing grain. Grain is very heavy and can easily crush a person who becomes entrapped in just a matter of a few seconds. This is particularly of concern when an individual enters a grain bin while it is being emptied of its contents. An auger in the bottom of the bin is used to remove the grain, by pulling the grain toward the center and the bottom of the bin. It is easy for an individual to become caught in the descending grain and be "sucked down" in much the same manner as when one is caught in quicksand.

Often the grain will "bridge over" as it is being removed from below. As one enters the grain bin and steps on what appears to be a solid grain mass, the bridge caves in, taking the person with it. Not only is suffocation likely, but the individual can get tangled in the machinery removing the grain. Care must be taken so that clothing, as well as hands, legs, and fingers, do not get caught in the drive systems of this machinery.

If it is necessary for an individual to enter the grain bin for some reason, several safety procedures are necessary. Not only must the auger be stopped, but the electrical switch must be locked and the operating key removed. A safety harness should be worn whenever entering a grain storage bin or silo. It is also wise to have a coworker present who is trained in appropriate rescue techniques. Coworkers and family members should be informed whenever an individual is working around a grain silo on a farm.

Care should be taken when grain becomes stuck to storage facility walls. Often the farmer will enter a bin for the purpose of knocking this grain loose. This dangerous procedure can result in an avalanche of grain coming down and smothering the person. The Occupational Safety and Health Administration recommends that a person never enter grain bins under these circumstances.[6]

A rescue device that can help extricate trapped persons in flowing grain has been designed and is now in widespread use. This device is a rescue tube. It can be inserted into grain around an entrapped person, relieving the grain pressure on the individual.

The Occupational Safety and Health Administration (OSHA) has published grain handling standards. They call for the training of employees who are involved in the handling of all types of grain. Also there should be development of safe entry plans for grain bins. These plans must be shared with employees. Emergency plans, rescue procedures, and the presence of available rescue equipment are now required at grain storage facilities.

Lack of Ventilation

Improper ventilation of a grain storage bin or silo can result in a buildup of carbon dioxide which depletes the level of oxygen. Suffocation will occur very quickly when an individual enters such a silo where there is a lack of adequate oxygen. Similar dangerous buildups of nitrogen may also occur in facilities where silage treated with high levels of nitrogen fertilizers is being stored.

Any time it is necessary to enter a silo, regardless of what is being stored, it is important to make sure that there is an adequate supply of oxygen. This can be done by making sure that there is proper ventilation bringing in outside air. It is important to test the atmosphere for the presence of combustible gases and toxic agents on a regular basis. Also, all equipment used in the grain storage facilities should be routinely inspected to assure that it is in safe operating condition.

Exposure to Toxic Gases

Animal manure that is stored in enclosures without adequate oxygen produces poisonous gases. The buildup of these gases often occurs in manure waste pits and tanks. A manure waste pit is a confined space that has inadequate ventilation. The decomposition and fermentation of waste creates a toxic oxygen deficient atmosphere.[7] Although asphyxiation can occur at any time, hot and humid weather provide optimal conditions biologically for the increased generation of these toxic gases.

At least four toxic gases are present in these kinds of situations: carbon dioxide, ammonia, hydrogen sulfide, and methane. Fatality can result from actual exposure to the toxic gas or as the result of working in a confined, oxygenless environment.

Carbon dioxide displaces the oxygen that is needed by humans for proper body functioning. Without adequate oxygen for just a short period of time, humans will die. Ammonia can injure the eyes and the tissues of the respiratory system, particularly the lungs. Hydrogen sulfide, which has an odor of rotten eggs, can cause headaches, dizziness, and nausea. In a very short period of time paralysis of the diaphragm may result, eventually causing death. Methane, a highly flammable nontoxic gas, can cause headaches and will ignite easily causing serious injury and death.

Much of the work done to repair engines or equipment on farms is performed in enclosed spaces, such as in the barn, the tractor shed, or the garage. Often, particularly if the work is being performed during the winter months, the doors and windows are closed. The running of any kind of engine in an enclosed area with improper ventilation and without exhaust escape mechanisms can result in a buildup of carbon monoxide. Whenever an individual works on an engine that is running indoors, it is vital that fresh air be circulating in the area. Such adequate movement of air depends upon a forced ventilation system. Should a person be overcome by carbon monoxide, quick and effective emergency care procedures must be known and implemented immediately. The first thing that should be done is to leave the enclosed area and go outside where there is adequate oxygen. If a person becomes unconscious and is not breathing, someone must remove the individual to a place where there is clear air and begin giving CPR.

Danger of Chemicals

More than a billion pounds of pesticides are used in the United States each year. There are about 600 pesticides in use, and only 200 have been subjected to health standards.[8]

Hundreds of chemicals are used in the agricultural workplace. Insecticides, herbicides, fungicides, acids, alkalis, solvents, fertilizers, and food additives are common to farming operations throughout the nation. These various toxic substances can be very damaging to anyone coming into contact with them.

Special care must be taken when working with fertilizers and pesticides, particularly when using organophosphate insecticides and ammonia fertilizers. Ammonia, a colorless gas at ordinary temperatures, is used widely in fertilizers because it is effective in getting large amounts of nitrogen into the soil. Ammonia gas in the air irritates the lungs and can cause tissue damage. Contact with body surfaces can cause painful burns to the skin. Contact with the eyes can cause blindness in a very short time. Whenever farm workers use these kinds of fertilizers, water should be available in the field for emergency care purposes—as well as in kits worn by a worker handling the chemicals.

A number of measures should be taken whenever working with pesticides. Pesticides—chemicals used to kill rodents and insects—are toxic and in sufficient amounts can injure or kill an individual. The chemical names of the active ingredients of the agent used, the specific antidotes recommended, and the proper emergency care measures should be known by every person working with these agents.

As when using any toxic agent, the instructions for proper application should be known and followed carefully, especially the appropriate dosage. In addition, when handling these toxic agents the individual should wear proper equipment to protect against toxin contact with the skin. Gloves and long-sleeve jackets or shirts should be worn to protect the hands and the arms. Goggles always should be worn to protect the eyes.

Under provisions of federal legislation, any newly manufactured pesticide must undergo extensive testing and documentation of its effects before it can be marketed for general public use. Once approved, the pesticide container must have a label which includes warnings about the level of toxicity, instructions regarding application, and the type of protective clothing and equipment needed for individuals applying the chemical.

The Federal Insecticide, Fungicide, and Rodenticide Act classifies all pesticides into one of two groups: general use or restricted use. *General-use pesticides* are those that can be bought and used by anyone. They can be used safely without special application knowledge, as long as the instructions on the label are followed.

Restricted-use pesticides can only be applied by persons who have met certain training standards for handling the particular substances. These substances have potential for serious adverse effects if they are not properly applied. They contain ingredients suspected of causing general illnesses, skin disorders, chronic bronchitis, or which even may be carcinogenic.

It is necessary to certify pesticide applicators who work with such restricted use pesticides. State agriculture departments have the responsibility for certifying individuals who can purchase and handle restricted use substances. Certification requires training in the handling of chemicals, calibration of sprayers, disposal of containers, and having

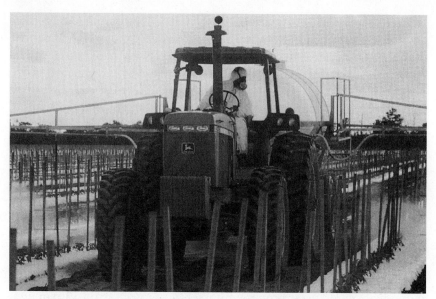

When applying pesticides, the agricultural worker must wear appropriate personal protective equipment—gloves, clothing, and head gear.

an understanding of the effect of the chemical on the environment. Periodic recertification is mandated. Two distinct certification groups have been identified: private and commercial. Farmers and ranchers meet the private applicator classification.

In 1994 a new worker protection standard issued by the Environmental Protection Agency went into effect. This standard requires compliance with product label instructions for all pesticide uses, including compliance from those working on small family farms.

Equipment used to apply pesticides should be cleaned before storage, and the pesticides should be stored in the original containers in a location where they cannot be spilled accidentally. Empty cans should be disposed of in a safe and proper manner. They should not be left lying around the barn, the yard, or the shed. As with any poisonous substance, pesticides should be kept away from children. This is no easy task when children often spend a great amount of time playing around the buildings on a farm.

Electrocution and Electrical Shock

The agricultural worker is exposed to numerous situations in which electrical shock or electrocution may result. These circumstances may result from work about the house, in the farm buildings, and in the fields. Agriculture workers must have a basic understanding of electrical wiring, electrical circuits, insulation, and grounding procedures. Any electrical work that is performed by the farmer must meet national, state, and local codes and regulations. For this reason, the person doing any kind of electrical repair or installation work must be familiar with all code regulations and have knowledge in application of the principles of electricity.

Proper grounding of all electrical circuits is necessary to protect against electrical shock. A grounding plug should be used whenever electrical tools, heaters, and electrical motors are being used.[9]

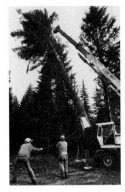

Forestry is one of the most dangerous types of employment, resulting in many fatalities and disabling injuries each year.

Care must always be taken when operating farm machinery to protect against contact with overhead power lines. It is possible for large machines, such as cornpickers and grain augers, as well as aluminum ladders and radio antennas, to make contact with power lines and become a dangerous conductor of electrical power. Individuals operating a tractor or other farm machinery, should make every effort to move machinery away from power lines.

Safety Concerns in Other Rural Occupations

Many employees work in rural settings that are not associated with agriculture. As with any occupation there are specific risk factors for fatality, injury, and disability. It is impossible within the context of this chapter to examine every occupation that is principally carried out in the nonurban setting. However, forestry is an example that merits special attention here.

Forestry is one of the most dangerous types of employment in the United States. The death rate among those employed in cutting trees is more than 160 per 100,000 full-time forestry employees.[10] A variety of conditions common to logging result not only in fatalities, but in serious injury and disability. Trees falling on the victim is reported in nearly half of all logging related deaths.[11]

Forestry involves the use of dangerous types of machinery, including mechanized saws and chain saws. Each of these can cause injury. The vibration and noise accompanying the use of chain saws is a risk factor for injury among loggers. Logging also is a physically demanding type of employment. Fatigue and inattention often contribute to fatal or injury-producing circumstances.

Often the person employed in logging has to ascend into the trees to carry out the cutting process. This necessitates the use of safety harnesses, although falls resulting in serious disabling injuries still are common.

Usually logging takes place in isolated localities in the forests, along fire lanes or logging trails deep in the woods. This means when an injury occurs, rather lengthy periods of time may pass before proper emergency care can be obtained. Access to the injured person by emergency vehicles is often hindered since work is not occurring along easily traversed roadways. Such factors contribute to the condition and future prognosis of the injured individual.

As is true in all occupational settings, careful preventive measures are paramount. Among loggers involved in the forestry industry continuing education, use of safety equipment, and the availability of emergency care equipment at the scene of the work is always necessary.

Summary

Although to an outsider the rural agricultural setting may appear tranquil and safe, farming, ranching, and other rural industries are dangerous occupations. Based on fatality rates, agriculture is one of the most hazardous occupational groupings. In addition many disabling injuries occur to agricultural workers every year.

Modern farming necessitates the use of highly mechanized kinds of machinery. Many injuries, as well as fatalities, occur each year involving the use of this type of equipment. Whether unclogging a moving machine or making minor repairs with an engine running, individuals risk serious injury when around mechanized equipment.

Tractors are the most commonly used piece of farm machinery; they also account for far too many fatalities and injuries. Commonly, tractor accidents result from turnovers. Rollover protective structures (ROPS) and the use of seat belts while operating tractors have been shown to be effective in reducing the possibility of injury or death. Alert operation, in the fields and on the roads and highways, is necessary to prevent fatalities and injuries while operating a tractor.

Numerous other situations lead to injuries and fatalities in rural settings. Extensive injuries have been associated with the improper use of pesticides; the same danger potential applies to working around grain storage bins. In every instance the worker must be alert and take preventive measures to reduce the incidence of injury and death. In this way agricultural work will be fulfilling and can contribute to a safe and enjoyable life-style.

There are other types of employment occurring principally in rural settings that present unique risks for injury. One of the most dangerous is forestry. Individuals involved in logging are faced with a number of situations that have caused death and injury to thousands. These dangers can only be reduced with careful attention to the risks and to the practice of preventive measures.

Discussion Questions

1. Using data indicate the extent of danger involved in working in an agricultural setting.
2. Discuss some of the factors that result in injury and fatality among rural populations.
3. Do you feel that the Occupational Safety and Health Act standards should be applied to all agricultural workers? Explain your answer.
4. What are the provisions of the Field Sanitation Standard?
5. What are the most common types of accidents that occur in connection with the use of farm machinery?
6. What are the major causes of tractor-related injuries and fatalities?
7. What is a ROPS?
8. When should a child be permitted to accompany the driver on a tractor? Explain your answer.
9. Discuss some of the dangers of grain bin storage.
10. What are some of the dangers associated with gases that build up in manure storage tanks?
11. What are some of the toxic chemicals a farmer is likely to contact in the process of carrying out the various tasks of farming?
12. Explain the differences between general use and restricted use classification of pesticides.
13. Identify measures that need to be taken to protect against electrocution in the agricultural setting.
14. What are some of the risk factors associated with the forestry industry of logging?
15. Identify other types of industries principally found in rural localities and discuss safety concerns unique to each.

Suggested Readings

Avers, Laura. "A, B, Cs are Elementary to Farm Rescue Workers," *Ohio Monitor* 64, no. 9 (September 1991): 4–9.

Barker, Teresa H. "When the Trees Fall, Make Sure the Fallers Stand," *Safety and Health* 146, no. 3 (September 1992): 44–47.

Centers for Disease Control and Prevention. "Fatalities Attributed to Entering Manure Waste Pits—Minnesota, 1992," *Morbidity and Mortality Weekly Report* 42, no. 17 (7 May 1993): 325–28.

Elkind, Pamela Dee. "Correspondence between Knowledge, Attitudes, and Behavior in Farm Health and Safety Practices," *Journal of Safety Research* 24, no. 3 (Fall 1993): 171–79.

Elliott-Proctor, Brenda. "The Tragic Harvest," *Ohio Monitor* 64, no. 9 (September 1991): 10–17.

Etherton, John R., and others. "Agricultural Machine-Related Deaths," *American Journal of Public Health* 81, no. 6 (June 1991): 766–68.

Geddes, Annmarie L. "Deadly Shelter," *Ohio Monitor* 64, no. 9 (September 1991): 18–21.

Goodman, Richard A., and others. "Fatalities Associated with Farm Tractor Injuries: An Epidemiologic Study," *Public Health Reports* 100, no. 3 (May–June 1985): 329–33.

Helgerson, Steven D., and Samuel Milham. "Farm Workers Electrocuted When Irrigation Pipes Contact Powerlines," *Public Health Reports* 100, no. 3 (May–June 1985): 325–28.

Heyer, Nicholas J., and others. "Occupational Injuries Among Minors Doing Farm Work in Washington State: 1986 to 1989," *American Journal of Public Health* 82, no. 4 (April 1992): 557–60.

O'Connor, Thomas A., and others. "Agricultural Injury Surveillance Using a State Injury Registry," *Journal of Safety Research* 24, no. 3 (Fall 1993): 155–66.

Rook, Martin. "ROPS: No Tractor Should Be Without One," *Ohio Monitor* 60, no. 11 (November 1987): 14–15.

Slappendel, Carol, and others. "Factors Affecting Work-Related Injury Among Forestry Workers: A Review," *Journal of Safety Research* 24, no. 1 (Spring 1993): 19–32.

Stoskopf, Carleen H., and Veen, Jonathan. "Farm Accidents and Injuries: A Review and Ideas for Prevention," *Journal of Environmental Health* 47, no. 5 (March–April, 1985): 250–52.

Thurber, Sarah. "Farmers Face Four Growing Hazards," *Safety and Health* 149, no. 4 (April 1994): 50–54.

Endnotes

1. Unless otherwise noted, statistical data in this chapter are from National Safety Council, *Accident Facts, 1993 Edition* (Itasca, IL: National Safety Council, 1993).
2. Ibid., 34.
3. Ibid., 107.

4. Martin Rook, "ROPS: No Tractor Should Be Without One," *Ohio Monitor* 60, no. 11 (November 1987): 14.
5. Brenda Elliott-Proctor, "The Tragic Harvest," *Ohio Monitor* 64, no. 9 (September 1991): 15.
6. Annmarie L. Geddes, "Deadly Shelter," *Ohio Monitor* 64, no. 9 (September 1991): 18–21.
7. Centers for Disease Control and Prevention, "Fatalities Attributed to Entering Manure Waste Pits—Minnesota, 1992," *Morbidity and Mortality Weekly Report* 42, no. 17 (7 May 1993): 326–27.
8. Sarah Thurber, "Farmers Face Four Growing Hazards," *Safety and Health* 149, no. 4 (April 1994): 52.
9. Further discussion of electricity and concerns related to electrocution is found in chapter 2.
10. National Institute for Occupational Safety and Health, "Logging Fatalities in the United States," *Farm Safe 2000* (Winter 1993): 6.
11. Ibid.

CHAPTER 7

The Motor Vehicle—Necessity and Potential Hazard

Chapter Outline

Introduction
Accident Statistics
Causes of Motor Vehicle Crashes
   Human Factors
   Age Factors
   Vehicular Factors
   Environmental Factors
Motor Vehicle Operation and Alcohol Use
   Physiology of Drinking
   Effects of Alcohol on Driving
   Driving Under the Influence
   Public Policy and Alcohol-Related Crashes
Motor Vehicle Collisions
Impact Restraints
   Active Restraints—Seat Belts
   Passive Restraints
Speed Limits
Pedestrian Safety
Safety at Rail Crossings
Summary
Discussion Questions
Suggested Readings
Endnotes

Introduction

Throughout history various inventions have profoundly changed the course of human life. Without the invention of the wheel, civilization's increasingly mobile lifestyles would have been unthinkable. Development of the printing press stimulated an unprecedented flow of ideas and knowledge. Hundreds of other innovations, perhaps most recently the microchip, have had significant impacts upon the world in which we live. The development of the motor vehicle or "horseless carriage" is one such invention that has played a major role in revolutionizing human life during the past century.

The motor vehicle and related technology are at the core of the economic structure of much of the world today. They are major factors in the manufacturing economy of the United States, Japan, and Germany. The economy of most of the nations of the Middle East rides on the world's need for oil to propel motorized vehicles. If the automotive industry becomes depressed, so does much of the rest of the U.S. economy. If a labor dispute closes down a major sector of the automotive industry, the effect is soon felt among hundreds of related industries. If the price of new cars goes up, the entire American economy is similarly affected by inflation. In the United States many households cannot function without more than one motor vehicle; many families have several automobiles. In addition, for hundreds of thousands of Americans such as truck drivers, traveling sales persons, and public transportation workers, the motor vehicle is the basic means of employment.

The motor vehicle has changed the lifestyles of the citizens of most nations of the world. This is dramatically noted among the population residing in the industrialized nations. The automobile has enabled everyone in the 1990s to be more mobile than were their great-grandparents. At the beginning of the twentieth century one's mobility was often limited to a short horse and buggy trip to the nearest town or village. Today it is not unusual to drive several hundred miles in one day for purposes of carrying out one's work, for recreational activities, or to visit family members.

Development of expansive highway systems has changed the landscape of most nations in the past half-century. The federal interstate highway system in the United States has cut "ribbons of highways" through urban communities, across rich farmland, over mountain ranges, and into areas of the country never before penetrated by public roads. Nearly every metropolitan urban community is crisscrossed by expressway systems that permit thousands of motor vehicles to move in and out of cities traveling at high rates of speed. Suburban communities, as well as small rural towns, are within easy reach of the many services available in large urban settings.

The horseless carriage of today is an efficient, fuel-consuming machine. The need for gasoline to run the millions of motor vehicles in the United States and throughout the globe has focused increased attention on those regions where oil is drilled, processed, and sold. Much of the world—particularly the United States, Japan, and much of

Europe—have become economically and politically dependent on imported oil. These factors have had significant impact in changing the political and economic structures of many countries since the early 1970s.

While it plays a major role in improving the life of people throughout the world, the motor vehicle also has brought with it an influx of problems. The internal combustion engine gives off a number of gases that cause pollution which contaminates the environment. These gases can cause decay, kill vegetation, and negatively impact the health of many people.

In spite of the ever improving efficiency of motor vehicles and the extensive roadway systems, thousands of fatalities and injuries occur annually as the result of motor vehicle collisions. Even though measures for improving the safe operation of motor vehicles have been the focus of a number of different community agencies since the introduction of the first horseless carriages, motor vehicle safety should be the concern of every individual—whether a motor vehicle operator, motor vehicle passenger, or pedestrian.

Accident Statistics

Motor vehicle accidents are the leading cause of death in the United States for persons between the ages of 1 and 24. They are responsible for more deaths than the next four causes combined among those of college age.

Slightly more than 40,000 persons die each year from injuries sustained in motor vehicle collisions.[1] If that figure is difficult to comprehend, drive through a town of that size and imagine the ramifications if every resident were to be killed in the next 12 months.

The first recorded automobile fatality occurred in 1899 in New York City when a man who stepped off a streetcar was struck by an automobile. He was pronounced dead shortly afterward.[2] Since that first incident in 1899, more than 2 million people have lost their lives as a result of motor vehicle crashes. More lives have been lost in the United States from motor vehicle crashes than have died in all of the wars in the nation's history from the time of the American Revolution to the Persian Gulf War and the conflict in Somalia.

Motor vehicle crashes result not only in fatalities but they are responsible for many disabling injuries and much economic loss as well. Approximately 2.2 million disabling injuries were reported in the United States from motor vehicle collisions in one recent year.[3] The economic cost of all motor vehicle crashes was estimated at more than $156 billion in that same year—a figure that includes related

> **HEALTH OBJECTIVES FOR THE NATION, YEAR 2000 MOTOR VEHICLES**
>
> 1. Reduce motor vehicle crash fatalities.
> 2. Reduce alcohol-related motor vehicle crash fatalities.
> 3. Increase use of occupant protection systems, such as seat belts, automatic crash protection, and child safety seats.
>
> Source: Department of Health and Human Services, *Healthy People 2000: National Health Promotion and Disease Prevention Objectives,* 1991.

medical expenses, insurance costs, wages lost as the result of injuries suffered, and related property damage.

The need for reducing the numbers of fatalities from motor vehicle crashes was noted by the Department of Health and Human Services in the development of health objectives for the nation.[4] A reduction of 20 percent in fatalities due to motor vehicle collisions by the year 2000 was established. In order to achieve this objective, three specific population groups were targeted for special program emphasis: children under 14 years of age, young people between 15 and 24, and senior citizens.

Causes of Motor Vehicle Crashes

There are many different causes of motor vehicle crashes. Usually more than one specific cause is identified for any given incident.

Human Factors

Of the many possible causes, the human factor is of primary importance. Most listings of the cause of vehicular collisions indicate some relationship to the driver. The driver may have been cited for drunken driving. The crash may have been the result of the driver's losing control of the vehicle or of excessive speeding. The motor vehicle operator may have been operating the car or van in a careless manner.

Errors in judgment have been identified as major causes of motor vehicle crashes. The failure to abide by rules of appropriate driving is considered human failure. Such rules include driving within posted speed limits, yielding the right of way when appropriate, and passing with caution. Many times fatigue, drowsiness, lack of attention, and other human conditions precipitate a collision. Excessive speed implies failure to exercise good judgment by the driver; so does failure to follow traffic flow regulations. In addition, many motor vehicle crashes are the result of the lack of some specific driving skill. Consequently, the major focus of any motor vehicle crash reduction program must include educational activities that are designed to improve human driving attitudes and behavioral patterns.

Age Factors

Every age group is involved in motor vehicle crashes. However, nearly a third of all such occurrences involve males between the ages of 15 and 24. In spite of the fact that this is the age at which a young man is physically most alert, this is also the age at which risk-taking behaviors and peer group pressures are predominant. The possibility of death or disabling injury occurring is far removed from the consciousness of most adolescent and young adult males. Lack of judgment and inexperience contribute to the potential for becoming involved in a motor vehicle crash. Considering all of the physical, emotional, and social dimensions that come into play, effective measures must be designed to develop a safety consciousness in all individuals, particularly adolescent and young adult males.

Vehicular Factors

While the major focus of any motor vehicle crash reduction program should be designing activities to improve the human factor, it must be noted that a number of other factors are involved in motor vehicle crashes relating to the vehicle itself. How often does an accident seem to result from the driver's losing control when in reality a structural defect was responsible for the crash? Many motor vehicle crashes that appear to be the fault of improper driver behavior may have occurred because of some failure or defect in vehicle design or construction.

In assessing the various causes of crashes, often minimal attention is given to the design and construction of the vehicle itself. Numerous things can go wrong with a motor vehicle since it is made up of thousands of different interacting parts. Some flaws may be inherent in the manufacture of the vehicle; others may develop over time with use.

The basic structure of most motor vehicles is safer today than in the past. Overall, improved engineering and design have made for better constructed vehicles. Yet since the mid-1960s various motor vehicle recall campaigns also have taken place.

It is estimated that more than 150 million motor vehicles have undergone recalls in the past 30 years. These recall programs usually are initiated when consumers discover a problem and report it. Manufacturers themselves may take such action when they become aware of

> ## USE OF BOOSTER CABLES
>
> It is necessary to know how to properly use booster cables in starting a motor vehicle with a dead battery. One should never smoke or hold an open flame near a battery. Care must be taken to avoid cross-connection. Cross-connection may produce sparks and could cause an explosion.
>
> The vehicles involved in the process should not be touching. The ignition should be off in the disabled vehicle. The following sequence should occur:
>
> 1. Clamp the *positive charge* on the disabled vehicle first.
> 2. Then clamp the other *positive charge* to the battery of the nondisabled vehicle.
> 3. Clamp the *negative charge* to the battery of the good vehicle.
> 4. Finally, clamp the remaining *negative charge* to the battery of the disabled vehicle.
>
> Start the engine of the nondisabled vehicle. Once it is running, the driver in the disabled vehicle should turn the ignition and attempt to start that engine. Once the disabled engine is running, the clamps of the booster cables should be removed in the reverse order from which they were put in place.

a potentially dangerous part. Complaints of possible problems are reported to the National Highway Traffic Safety Administration. When a safety defect is identified, the manufacturer is required to notify owners of that particular model vehicle. The owner is requested to bring the vehicle into a local dealership and the manufacturer is required to make corrections at no charge to the customer.

Environmental Factors

There are 3.9 million miles of public roads in the United States.[5] The road and highway systems upon which motor vehicles are driven vary greatly. There are narrow two-lane country dirt and gravel roads with nothing separating oncoming vehicles. On paved two-lane roads only a mid-line marking separates passing motor vehicles. On the other hand, there are multilane expressways on which thousands of motor vehicles are operated at maximum speeds. No matter what the size, the road structure should be constructed so that the tires grip the roadway firmly in all kinds of weather. The shoulders alongside the roads should be constructed so that they do not contribute to an operator's losing control of the motor vehicle.

Many motor vehicle crashes result from abnormal road surface conditions. It is not unusual for road surfaces to be rough or for there

DRIVING IN COLD WEATHER CONDITIONS

In much of the northern part of the United States people must learn to adapt their driving skills to cope with snow, ice, and cold temperatures. For the inexperienced winter driver a half-inch of snow can cause serious problems. Yet, for those individuals who have developed cold weather driving skills, winter does not need to be frightening.

One must remember that braking distances are significantly increased when there is ice and snow on the roads. Normal braking distance under ideal conditions at 20 miles per hour is between 18 and 22 feet. With snow-packed and ice conditions this braking distance may be as long as 195 feet (the distance that one needs to brake under normal conditions at 60 miles per hour).

When braking on snow or ice the driver must learn to "squeeze" the brakes. This involves gently pressing the brake pedal down until you feel the wheels nearly lock. Release the brakes at this point and then squeeze the pedal down again. This procedure keeps the wheels rolling without locking.

When in a skid on ice and packed snow, the experienced driver has learned to turn the wheel in the direction of the skid. When skidding to the right, turn the wheel right; when skidding to the left, turn the wheel to the left.

During cold weather every driver should have several safety-related items available in the trunk of the vehicle. There should be a warm blanket, dry gloves, socks, hat, and coat. A shovel and sand will be helpful should one become stuck on the ice and snow. Everyone operating a motor vehicle must have an ice scraper to clean the windshield of ice and snow.

---

to be uneven breaks in the surfaces. In spite of road conditions and the vehicle design, the vehicle operator is expected to keep the motor vehicle under control at all times.

Existing road systems must be kept in safe condition so that motor vehicle crashes are not likely to occur. Roadways, as well as adjacent areas, must be efficient, effective, and as free of hazards as possible. Many factors are necessary in the development of a safe highway environment. One important cause of motor vehicle crashes resulting in death and injury is the presence of obstacles alongside the road. Telephone and electric poles, ditches, roadside signs, brick mail boxes, and trees are examples of such obstacles. Narrow bridges present another serious roadside hazard. In addition, road surfaces must be designed to prevent sliding and skidding.

Highway systems should be built only after extensive planning by safety engineers, highway consultants, law enforcement personnel, and other highway safety experts. Many features can be built into roads that make them safer. For example, guardrails can be constructed of impact-absorbing material and supports for traffic control devices can be engineered to yield or break away upon impact. Poles situated along the roadway should be constructed of aluminum rather than of concrete. Exit and entrance ramps for high-speed roads should not interfere with the flow of traffic. Wide shoulders should be constructed on each side of the road to provide a lane for performing emergency road services such as changing a tire. The road shoulders should be level with the roadway and should not be constructed of loose stones or gravel. The field of highway engineering provides many opportunities for creative engineering research and development.

Motor Vehicle Operation and Alcohol Use

Approximately one-half of all motor vehicle fatalities result from the use of alcohol. Most Americans believe it is socially acceptable to drink alcohol in moderation. Major problems arise, however, when the use of alcohol is accompanied with driving of motor vehicles. Intoxicated or alcohol-impaired drivers have been major concerns to safety, law enforcement, public health, and emergency medical care personnel for years. The carnage resulting from intoxicated drivers has become an increasing public policy concern throughout the nation. In an attempt to draw attention to the problem and to stimulate broad-range initiatives, the federal government in 1990 set a goal of reducing alcohol-related motor vehicle fatalities by more than 10 percent by the year 2000.[6]

Physiology of Drinking

A brief review of the physiology of alcohol consumption will aid in understanding why the consumption of a small amount of alcohol can hinder driving performance. Foods taken into the stomach go through a process known as *digestion*. However, this process does not occur when alcohol is consumed. Once alcohol has passed into the stomach, a process referred to as *absorption* takes place. Alcohol diffuses through the walls of the gastrointestinal tract where the tiny blood vessels pick up the alcohol and circulate it throughout the body by way of the bloodstream. Absorption occurs in the small intestine as well as in the stomach.

As alcohol is distributed throughout the body, it becomes diluted. The amount of alcohol in the blood is spoken of as the *blood-alcohol*

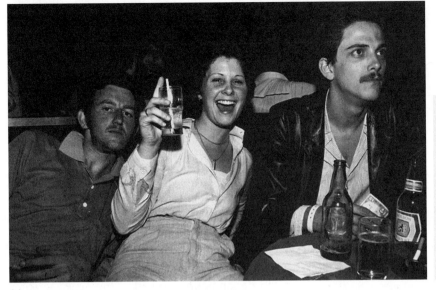
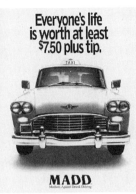

(a) (b)

(a) Drinking of alcoholic beverages is part of the social life of many Americans. (b) However, drinking and driving can result in serious injury and death. Mothers Against Drunk Driving is a volunteer organization that encourages people who drink to find alternative ways of getting home.

level or the *blood-alcohol concentration* (BAC). The effect of the alcohol on the behavioral patterns of an individual is related to the blood-alcohol concentration. The higher the BAC, the greater the functional impairment of the body. The moderate drinker may have a blood-alcohol level of only a few hundredths of one percent. Impairment begins when the BAC reaches a level from 0.03 to 0.10 percent. At this level feelings of relaxation and sedation are experienced. There is a steady decline in control of voluntary muscles involved in performance of fine motor skills. Functional impairment becomes serious when the BAC level is 0.10 percent or higher. Vision and hearing are affected as is judgment. There is a reduction in performance of gross motor skills. Profound intoxication is noted when the BAC level reaches 0.20 percent.

Effects of Alcohol on Driving

A number of important physiological effects of alcohol relate to motor vehicle driving. Alcohol affects the functioning of the brain; it depresses the brain so that an individual under the influence of alcohol is unable to make "normal" judgments. For example, vision becomes blurred and a condition known as "tunnel vision" often occurs—that is, peripheral vision becomes impaired. These initial effects of intoxication are followed by impairment of the reflexes and other normal reactions. Gross motor skills and judgment are impeded. Night-driving skills are impacted negatively.

The ingestion of as few as two beers in one hour can slow a person's reaction time by as much as two-fifths of a second. This may not seem significant. However, a vehicle going 60 miles an hour can travel 34 feet in this period of time. The potential for causing an injury producing collision or a fatality in such a situation becomes obvious.

Driving Under the Influence

Many different ideas, programs, laws, and initiatives have been proposed or implemented in an attempt to address the problem of driving under the influence of alcohol. It is estimated that 1.3 million drivers are arrested annually for driving while intoxicated or driving under the influence of alcohol.[7] Those arrested are dealt with in a variety of ways. The specific approach often depends upon whether the arrest is for a first offense or whether there has been a history of arrests for drunken driving. In some instances the individual is given a fine; in other situations the penalty may involve suspension of driving privileges for a period of time; and occasionally a jail sentence may be handed down by the court.

If problems associated with driving while intoxicated are to be solved, efforts must be made to get the person involved into some type of alcohol treatment program. A variety of educational countermeasures aimed at the problem of driving while intoxicated have been developed. Among the most common programs are education-information courses. These programs are designed to help those charged with driving while under the influence of alcohol to learn and understand the dangers of their behavior so that attitudes and behaviors can be changed.

As the individual in the education-information program learns about the effect of alcohol consumption on driving skills, it is hoped that the person will examine his or her own drinking behavior as it relates to driving. The basic concept is that the better educated people are about alcohol and driving, the less likely they will be to drink and drive. However, there is some question as to the effectiveness of such educational programs in combating driving-under-the-influence behavior patterns.

Another type of program that has been used in certain localities involves requiring adolescents convicted of driving under the influence to visit hospital emergency departments and morgues to observe the results of motor vehicle crashes. While at the hospital the individuals see the treatment of trauma cases and learn of associated medical problems in the particular situation. In addition to these mandated visits, educational sessions regarding alcohol and its effects on driving are given. Research has questioned the value of this type of program for long-term attitude improvement.[8] The ethics of infringing on the confidentiality of victims at the hospital emergency center also has been questioned.

Public Policy and Alcohol-Related Crashes

Though model education-information programs for individuals charged with driving under the influence of alcohol have some place as an alcohol countermeasure, resolution to the problem also must include other initiatives. Numerous public policy actions have been designed throughout the country for the purpose of reducing alcohol-related motor vehicle crashes.

Laws Relating to Driving-Under-the-Influence

In the past decade more than 700 state and local laws have been passed stiffening the penalty for driving while under the influence of alcohol.[9] For example, in Massachusetts a mandatory ten-year license revocation, minimum one-year prison sentence, and fine are the penalty when an individual is convicted of vehicular homicide while driving under the influence of alcohol. In California a BAC of 0.10 percent is now punishable by law and is taken as *prima facie* evidence for driving under the influence. In another state, Alabama, suspension of a drivers' license is now mandatory upon a person's first conviction for driving under the influence of alcohol. Suspension time is increased for subsequent convictions.[10]

In Michigan a minimum mandatory 30-day license suspension is required upon first-time conviction for operating a motor vehicle under the influence of liquor or drugs.[11] Also, drivers who fail or refuse to take a blood-alcohol chemical test will have their licenses confiscated by police. A driver will receive points against his or her driver's record if open intoxicants are found in the automobile.

Administrative license revocation (ALR) has become the law in more than half of the states. The goal of administrative license revocation (ALR) is to remove drunk drivers from the road. ALR refers to either the revocation or suspension of a driver's license before conviction for all alcohol-related offenses. Law enforcement personnel may revoke or suspend the license of drivers who fail or refuse a blood-alcohol chemical test. The actual license can be confiscated by law enforcement personnel at the time of the arrest.

Minnesota was the first state with ALR provisions.[12] The specific provisions of ALR legislation vary among the states. In California police are allowed to take the license of a motorist who fails or refuses to take a blood, breath, or urine test for alcohol. In Nevada an individual's refusal to take a BAC test at the request of a police officer can result in the loss of the driver's license immediately. There is evidence that in states with administrative license revocation provisions there tends to be a reduction in motor vehicle crashes.[13]

There are groups and individuals who have challenged these provisions on constitutional grounds—i.e., violation of one's civil rights. However, such legislation has been strongly supported by Mothers Against Drunk Driving (MADD), the National Highway Traffic Safety Administration, the National Safety Council, as well as many automobile insurance companies.

About half of the states permit license suspension for drivers with BAC levels above 0.10 percent from the time of their arrest until the trial. In some jurisdictions prison is now mandatory on the second offense. Penalties for refusal to submit to BAC testing at police sobriety checkpoints are now implemented in some locations. Stiffer fines, suspension of drivers' licenses, jail sentences for repeated offenders, and jail sentences for those involved in traffic accidents resulting in injury or fatality are other actions implemented by certain state and local governments.

Reduction of the BAC Level

It is the opinion of many safety and law enforcement professionals that lowering the legal blood-alcohol concentration level (BAC) would remove many potentially dangerous drivers from the roads and highways who now operate motor vehicles. In most states the legal BAC level for determining that an individual is driving under the influence is 0.10. Five states have lowered their BAC level for determination of intoxication of drivers to 0.08. There is increasing support to have state legislation passed to reduce the BAC level to at least 0.08 nationally, and even lower levels are recommended by some safety professionals. As one can suspect, the liquor industry has opposed all initiatives to lower these standards.

Implied Consent Laws

An issue related to the discussion of BAC levels is whether drivers should be required to submit to BAC testing. Should an individual stopped on *suspicion* of driving under the influence of alcohol be required to take a BAC test? Should *random testing* be carried out for all drivers on public roadways? Many people have suggested that such mandated BAC testing is an infringement of individual rights and as a result should not be permitted.

Implied consent laws require that a driver must automatically agree to a breath test whenever a law enforcement officer has reason to believe that the individual is driving under the influence of alcohol. In states with implied consent laws, if an individual refuses to take the test, the driver's license may be suspended immediately.

Some states and communities have implemented random breath-testing programs. Such programs might be effective in reducing problems associated with drunken driving. The risk of being stopped at a police sobriety checkpoint can be an effective countermeasure in reducing the number of persons driving while intoxicated.[14] Sobriety checkpoints are conducted by law enforcement officers at which drivers are stopped at random and evaluated for alcohol use. If behaving suspiciously, drivers can be required to have their blood-alcohol levels tested.

These types of alcohol countermeasures usually are not very strongly supported by the general public. Those who do not use alcohol are particularly opposed to being randomly stopped while driving. Whether such actions are an infringement of individual rights is open to question in the minds of many. In 1990 the United States Supreme Court ruled that sobriety checkpoints are not an infringement of individual rights. As a result many local jurisdictions have continued to use sobriety checkpoints in an attempt to reduce the incidence of driving while intoxicated. These activities are conducted in some communities on a regular basis. In other localities they occur on special occasions, such as New Years Eve, on certain holidays, or at times when it is known that parties are being held at which alcohol is likely to be present, such as graduation parties or homecoming parties at colleges and universities.

The Legal Drinking Age

What age should be considered minimum in order to be able to drink? During the early 1970s over half of the states lowered their minimum drinking age from 21 to 18 and 19. It was the position of many young adults that if they were old enough to vote, to enter the military service, and be considered as adults for other matters at 18, it should be acceptable for them to drink legally at this time in their lives.

In the early 1980s there was increasing movement and political pressure for states to reverse these earlier actions and raise the legal minimum drinking ages. This pressure was brought to bear by public interest groups or citizen activist groups concerned about the problem of alcohol and motor vehicle accident causation. Several governmental and official professional statements supported the need to raise minimum drinking ages. The National Transportation Safety Board (1982), the National Council on Alcoholism (1982), the Presidential Commission on Drunk Driving (1983), and the American Medical Association (1986) were examples of such groups issuing statements on this matter.

In 1984 the U.S. Congress passed the Uniform Minimum Drinking Age Act which required the federal Department of Transportation to withhold federal highway funds from any states that did not have a minimum drinking age of 21. Some individuals viewed this federal government action as "blackmail." Every state relies heavily upon federal funds for monies to build and repair their federal as well as state roadways. As a result, states virtually were *forced* to increase the minimum drinking ages. In 1988 Wyoming became the last state to raise the legal drinking age to 21, making all states now in compliance with the federal law.

This federal legislation and subsequent action of each state has not been without controversy. Some research evidence supports the contention that there has been a reduction of fatalities resulting from drunken driving among the 18- to 21-year-old age group.[15] Also, the higher drinking age is associated with lower rates of traffic crash involvement.[16] On the other hand, many disagree and feel that these laws are unnecessary and even an infringement of individual rights. The United States Supreme Court refused to support an appeal declaring the federal legislation to be unconstitutional.

Third-Party Responsibility

An increasing number of court decisions and local ordinances have held that individuals who sell, serve, or provide alcoholic beverages to a person who then commits an alcohol-related offense while driving is liable for damages incurred. These laws are known as *dram shop laws.*

One of the earliest court decisions occurred in 1984 in New Jersey when that state's supreme court ruled that a host could be held liable if liquor was served to a guest who subsequently caused injuries to others in a motor vehicle accident. Other courts have extended liability to employers who provide alcoholic beverages to minors. Tavern owners, bartenders, and those who directly serve the alcoholic drinks have been found to be legally responsible. Also, hosts of private parties have been held legally liable in several instances.

These legal developments have led to numerous changes in the operation of facilities which serve alcoholic beverages. For example, bartenders and those who serve alcoholic beverages such as waiters and waitresses now often undergo training to intervene with and not serve individuals who are already intoxicated. More specific procedures are taken to check identification cards for legal drinking age of clients. Staff are encouraged to offer food and/or water to those who might be intoxicated. Liability insurance premiums have risen dramatically or coverage is not even available in some localities for operators of facilities which serve alcoholic beverages.

Surgeon General's Workshop on Drunk Driving

In 1988 the Office of the United States Surgeon General held a workshop focusing on the problems associated with drunken driving. Among the many recommendations that resulted from this initiative were several that called for an all-out attack on alcohol consumption and driving.[17] One recommendation called for curbing the advertising of alcoholic beverages, particularly on college campuses. Since the minimum drinking age is 21 in all 50 states, it seems inappropriate to permit such advertising on campuses where the majority of students are under this age. The Surgeon General's Workshop also recommended that there should be a ban on the use of celebrities in beer and wine advertisements that appeal to youth.

The Surgeon General's Workshop on Drunk Driving also strongly supported the idea that athletic events and other youth-oriented activities should not be sponsored by alcoholic beverage companies. The workshop went so far as to recommend that antialcohol advertising

---

RECOMMENDATIONS OF THE PRESIDENTIAL COMMISSION ON DRUNK DRIVING

1. Raise legal drinking age to 21.
2. Admit victim's impact statement in court.
3. Use larger portions of fines for local alcohol programs.
4. Lower BAC required as proof of drunkenness.
5. Mandate that first offenders driving under the influence receive jail sentences or license suspensions.
6. Police should be permitted to carry out preliminary breath tests at the scene of an accident.
7. Make a person who sells alcoholic beverages to intoxicated individuals liable.
8. Provide restitution to victims of accidents involving drinking and driving.

Source: Surgeon General's Workshop on Drunk Driving, *Proceedings,* 1988.

should be encouraged to counter the advertising of alcoholic beverages. It was indicated that warning labels should be displayed when a beer or wine is shown on television.

Motor Vehicle Collisions

When a moving motor vehicle strikes another object, be it stationary or moving, a collision has occurred. Damage usually results to the various external parts of the vehicle. A fender may be dented, the hood damaged, or any number of things may take place that either makes the car inoperable or damages the appearance and basic structure of the vehicle.

The initial impact of the vehicle with whatever it hit is referred to as the *first collision*. Almost instantly, a *second collision* takes place. This is due to the forward momentum of the occupants in the vehicle. Occupants continue to move forward after the initial collision until contact is made with the internal structure of the car. The impact can be with a window, door, roof, front seat, steering wheel, or dashboard. It is this second collision that causes fatalities and serious injuries in motor vehicle crashes. Unless the driver or other occupants of the vehicle are restrained, forward motion will not stop until the individual has struck some interior object or has been thrown from the vehicle and struck some object outside, such as the ground, a tree, or the roadway pavement.

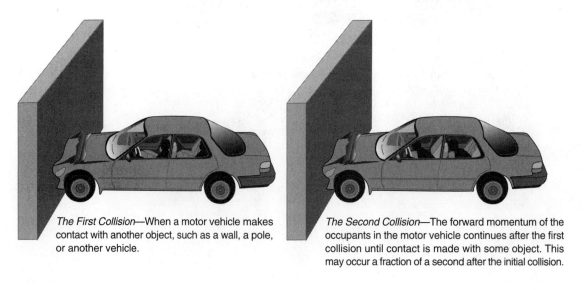

The First Collision—When a motor vehicle makes contact with another object, such as a wall, a pole, or another vehicle.

The Second Collision—The forward momentum of the occupants in the motor vehicle continues after the first collision until contact is made with some object. This may occur a fraction of a second after the initial collision.

There is ample evidence that the human body can withstand tremendous stress of abrupt deceleration. Therefore, most people can survive a severe collision, assuming that they do not "fly" into contact with the vehicle structure or are not ejected from the motor vehicle. For this reason, measures must be built into all motor vehicles to prevent forward momentum from occurring after the initial impact of the collision. In addition, people must become aware of the importance of taking measures that will help to protect against the second collision.

Protection also can be provided through energy-absorbing interior structures. High-penetration-resistant windshields have proven to be effective in reducing injuries to the face while not increasing the risk of brain injury. Current research initiatives are attempting to develop a windshield that would help prevent serious face and scalp lacerations. Energy-absorbing steering systems, introduced nearly 30 years ago, have proven to be effective in saving lives and reducing injuries to occupants involved in motor vehicle crashes.

Impact Restraints

Impact restraint measures can be grouped into two basic categories: active and passive.

Active Restraints—Seat Belts

The measure that has received the most widespread attention for protecting motor vehicle occupants from the second collision has been the development, installation, and use of seat belts. The use of seat belts in motor vehicles was suggested as early as 1937.[18] Seat or lap belts were developed as the first passenger restraint for use in automobiles in the mid-1950s. Without seat belts the majority of collision injuries involve the head striking the windshield, the face and chest impacting the steering wheel and dashboard, and the body colliding with doors or the roof of the vehicle, or involve physical ejection from the vehicle.

For almost a decade seat belts were considered an "extra" with the purchase of a new vehicle. Not until 1964 did lap belts become standard equipment. Belts were usually installed in the two front-seat positions. At that time there were no federal mandates for installation and use of belts. However, several states passed laws mandating the installation of lap belts in the front seat before a motor vehicle could be sold. The automotive manufacturing companies, finding it difficult to produce vehicles with and without belts to meet differing state regulations, eventually standardized installation in all vehicles.

The lap belt did keep people from being ejected at initial impact. However, in spite of the fact that such devices were seen as being effective in reducing injuries and fatalities, injuries still occurred to those who wore the lap belts. Individuals often experienced abdominal injuries as well as injuries to the spinal column. Lap belts do not prevent the occupant from jackknifing upon impact and striking the front window or the dash. For this reason, the three-point belt system was developed with the lap and the shoulder belts permanently connected.

The federal government passed legislation in 1966 that mandated that lap belts and shoulder belts must be provided for the two front-seat positions.[19] Lap belts were required in all other seating positions. This legislation became effective in 1968.

In 1972 another federal standard became effective that required vehicles to have a buzzer-light warning system that became activated when the lap belt was not fastened. A red light on the dash came on and a buzzer sounded if the lap belt was not extended at least four inches from its normally stowed position. No passenger car was to be manufactured for sale in the United States without this buzzer warning system.

This warning system was easily circumvented. All people had to do was pull out the belt several inches and hook it on some object near the floor and the warning system would not be activated. As a result, slightly more than a year later another standard went into effect that required that the engine of a car could not be started until the safety-belt system was connected properly. This was known as the *interlock system.* The engine could not be started until the driver and occupant in the right-front seating position had locked their belts. If the right-front seat was occupied after the engine was running, a buzzer-light system would become activated. Public reaction to the interlock system was negative and the federal government eliminated the required interlock system on all new automobiles in 1975.

Mandated Seat-Belt-Use Legislation

Today all cars manufactured for sale in the United States must have lap and shoulder belts. Emphasis during the 1980s changed from federal legislation to a focus on state laws that would mandate the use of seat belts.

In 1985 New York State became the first state to pass a safety-belt-use law. Today mandatory belt-use laws are in effect in 42 states along with the District of Columbia. Most of these mandates require seat belt use for occupants of the front seat; several provide for both front- and rear-seat occupants. Enforcement of these mandatory

FOUR BASIC TYPES OF AUTOMATIC SEAT BELTS

1. Detachable nonmotorized three-point belts (lap and shoulder)
2. Nondetachable motorized two-point (shoulder) belts
3. Detachable motorized two-point belts
4. Detachable nonmotorized two-point belts

Source: Allan F. Williams, et al., "Use of Seatbelts in Cars with Automatic Belts," *Public Health Reports* 107, no. 2 (March/April 1992):185.

belt-use laws varies, with the majority being what is termed *secondary enforcement.* This means that the law can only be enforced if the individual is stopped for another violation. The motor vehicle cannot be stopped primarily for a seat belt violation. Only in 11 states can the driver be stopped and ticketed for a primary seat belt violation.[20]

Numerous studies have been conducted to ascertain the effectiveness of mandatory seat-belt-use laws. Usage patterns indicate that initially following passage of seat belt laws there is an increase in use. This is followed by substantial use decline after a few months.[21] A major reason for this decline is the perception of the public that the law is not being enforced. This is particularly noted in states where the enforcement is secondary.

In states with belt laws approximately 62 percent of occupants use belts.[22] The federal government has set 85 percent belt usage as a goal to be achieved by the year 2000.[23] It is felt that in order to achieve this objective all states currently with no mandatory seat belt legislation must develop such regulations.

Beginning in 1990, under the mandate of the National Highway Safety Administration, all cars must have automatic restraints—either seat belts that automatically fasten when a person enters or starts the motor vehicle or airbags. This mandate applies to all cars except vans, small trucks, and utility vehicles.

Child Restraints

Adult-sized seat belts are not effective in providing protection for small children. Approximately 1,000 children under five years of age are killed each year in motor vehicle crashes.[24] Also, about 65,000 injuries occur to infants and young children. It is estimated that the risk of death or serious injury could be reduced by 70 percent if child infant seats were used.[25]

Until a child weighs approximately 40 pounds and stands 40 inches tall, the adult lap and shoulder belt system will be of little use.

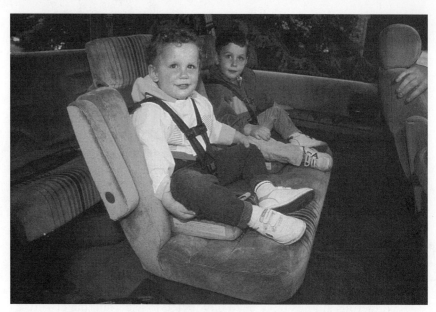

Every child should be placed in a safety seat when riding in a motor vehicle. All states have mandated child safety seat laws.

A sudden stop may thrust the infant or young child up and out of the belt system. Consequently, child restraint safety systems have been designed especially to provide protection for infants and young children.

Child safety seats must meet crash test requirements which have been established by the National Highway Transportation Safety Administration. The manufacturer must provide instructions for the proper installation of the seat.

These child safety seats keep children from being thrown into the windshield or dashboard or from being thrown about the vehicle following the initial collision. Standards have been issued for acceptable child restraint seats. They must fit the car, be easy to use, and be comfortable for the child. Infants up to 20 pounds should ride in infant-only seats which are placed backwards on the motor vehicle seat.

As with any preventive measure it is necessary for parents to place their children in these restraints. In 1978 the state of Tennessee became the first state to pass a mandatory child safety-seat law; now all 50 states have child safety-seat laws. In spite of these state mandates, many children are seen riding in motor vehicles without such safety restraints.

Often parents do not install the child safety seat properly. Other inappropriate practices include the use of seats that are too big for the age and size of the child. One of the most dangerous practices is for an adult to hold a child on his or her lap. This is particularly dangerous because in a collision the child can be easily thrown about the car or the adult may be thrust forward and crush the child against the dash and/or window.

Some people oppose the legal mandates for child safety seats on the grounds that they are expensive and that economically disadvantaged individuals cannot afford them. In many communities there are agencies that provide seats to those who cannot afford to purchase them. Many hospitals will not permit a parent to take a baby home unless there is a child safety seat in the motor vehicle.

An important question has been raised concerning parents who permit their children to ride in a motor vehicle without a child safety seat. Should such a child be killed in a collision, what is the legal responsibility of the parents? This question was addressed in a case in Florida in which a father was charged with homicide in the death of his child who was not in a seat belt. This individual was found guilty. Such a legal finding has very important ramifications for all adults driving with children in their motor vehicles.

Passive Restraints

Seat belt usage demands action on the part of the vehicle occupant. The individual must demonstrate active intent (hooking up the belt) for the device to be useful. Measures also have been developed that necessitate no active involvement by the vehicle occupant. Such protective mechanisms are called *passive restraints.* Certain passive devices have been required by federal standards since 1968—namely, the energy-absorbing steering column and windshield. Probably the most widely discussed passive safety device is the airbag.

Airbags

The airbag works on the concept that upon the initial impact of collision a device inflates so that those riding in the motor vehicle are provided with protective cushioning. The forward momentum of the occupants is absorbed by the inflated bag. The individual stays in contact with the bag so that impact with the front window, steering wheel, and dashboard does not occur.

Since airbags are effective only in head-on, frontal collisions, there is still a need to use seat and shoulder belts. Hence, airbags are designed to supplement, not replace, seat and shoulder belts. A major advantage of the airbag is that the force of the crash is distributed over a large portion of the person's body, whereas use of the lap and/or shoulder belt often results in extreme pressure where the belts touch the person.

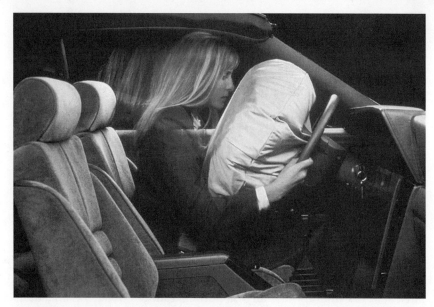

The airbag inflates within 1/20th of a second after a collision. When employed along with the shoulder and lap belt, the airbag is very effective in providing protection for the occupant from being thrown from, and about, the motor vehicle.

The airbag system becomes operational with forces equivalent to hitting a solid barrier at about 10 to 12 miles per hour. Sensors inside the bumpers or front end of the motor vehicle trigger the release of chemicals which inflate the bag within one-thirtieth of a second.[26] This system works when collisions are within 30 degrees of center. The airbag is concealed in the steering wheel hub and behind the dashboard and glove compartment. Deflation occurs when the vehicle returns to a controlled rate of movement.

Airbags do not provide protection in all collisions. For example, since the airbag gives protection only in a frontal impact collision, it is less effective in a chain reaction collision. The airbag is not designed to provide protection in a rear-end collision, a side impact crash, or a rollover.

There is little evidence that airbags might accidentally deploy under normal driving conditions. They are designed to operate only when a frontal collision occurs. There also is little evidence of an airbag failing to act when it is needed.

Experimentation with the airbag has taken place since the late 1950s. The first patent for an airbag was issued in 1953. Through the years different types of airbags have been designed, developed, and tested.

Research has shown that there are fewer upper body injuries where airbags have been deployed. However, they have no role to play in protecting against injuries to the lower extremities. Therefore, research has continued in an attempt to find ways to provide protection against injuries to the foot and lower leg where the brake and accelerator pedals are located. There also is need for stronger floors that would reduce floor crumbling in a crash. Airbags located in the auto foot well and in interior door panels have received increasing research interest. Airbags located in interior door panels would provide occupants with protection against side and rear-end crashes.

It must be acknowledged that airbags themselves can cause injuries. Facial abrasions and minor burns to the face and hands have been reported. This, however, must be considered minor compared to the value of the airbags in protecting against disabling or fatal injury.

Should state or national government mandate the installation of airbags in motor vehicles? This question has been discussed for years. Most automotive manufacturers have been opposed to federal mandates for airbags. They argue that there is doubt as to the effectiveness of the airbag and suggest the need for more definitive research. Economic factors have been another reason for opposition to the mandating of airbags in motor vehicles. It is estimated that airbags cost between $400 and $800 per motor vehicle.[27] This cost will be added to the price of the vehicle. As a result, consumers must become convinced of the value of the airbag passive restraint system to be willing to pay the extra costs involved.

Several times the federal Department of Transportation has issued regulations that would require new vehicles to have a passive airbag system. However, for a variety of reasons these deadlines have been modified and set back. For example, in 1984 government regulations were passed that all new cars must have passive restraints in front seats by the 1990 models. The manufacturers indicated they could not meet this deadline.

Current regulations are that by 1998 all new passenger cars must have dual front airbags to provide protection for the driver and front seat passenger. By 1999 all minivans and pickup trucks must have dual airbags. Several of the world's automobile manufacturers have announced they will equip all cars with airbags as standard equipment by the mid-1990s.

Individual purchasers of motor vehicles could provide a major impetus for the inclusion of airbags in the automotive manufacturing process if they were to demand that they be available on new vehicles. Should people become more safety conscious there would be less need for governmental mandate.

Other Passive Protective Measures

Other measures have been designed and are now installed as standard equipment in motor vehicles to protect the occupant from injury upon impact at the time of the second collision. Padded dashboards, safety-designed knobs and controls, and head restraints are now found in most automobiles. Federal standards require that motor vehicles be manufactured with energy-absorbing steering columns. These steering assemblies collapse in a collision and reduce the likelihood of serious injury resulting from the rear displacement of the steering assembly.

Energy-absorbing windshields also are built into motor vehicles. Laminated glass—a plastic core with glass bonded to it—is used in the construction of windshields. These windshields are designed to absorb some of the forward energy of the occupant. They have resulted in less severe facial injuries.

Speed Limits

In 1974, as an outgrowth of the recognized need to conserve energy, the federal government passed laws which lowered the maximum speed limits in the United States. Evidence was very clear that less fuel was consumed when driving at 50 to 55 miles per hour than at 60 to 70. To improve fuel conservation, maximum speed limits of 55 miles per hour were imposed on all open highways throughout the nation. This reduction of speed limits also had a positive effect on highway safety. Driving at slower speeds meant that the vehicle operator could maintain better control and that highway traffic flow would be more uniform.

In spite of the safety benefits of reduced speed limits, there were many who wanted speed limits returned to 65 miles per hour. Those who were particularly desirous of this were individuals and companies making their livelihood driving the nation's highways. The trucking industry was most active in pushing for change. As a result of such pressure, Congress passed the Surface Transportation and Uniform Relocation Act in 1987 which allowed states to increase speed limits on rural interstate highways from 55 to 65.

New Mexico became the first state to restore the 65-mile-per-hour speed limit. Most other states have taken such action, with only 8 retaining the 55-mile-per-hour limit.[28]

There seems to be evidence that this increase in speed limits has resulted in an increase in fatalities. There also is an increase in the actual driving speeds. Many motor vehicles are regularly clocked at speeds of 70 miles per hour or more. Even though the federal mandate was for travel on federal interstate highways there has been a noted increase in speeds on other roadways. One need only travel on an interstate highway in an urban community to realize that the change in speed limit did not affect just driving patterns on rural highways.

Pedestrian Safety

Many traffic fatalities involve individuals who are not riding in a motor vehicle. They involve people walking along the road, children running out into the traffic, and individuals entering the flow of traffic on foot for one reason or another. These kinds of situations are referred to as *pedestrian accidents.* Approximately 6,500 pedestrian fatalities occur annually.[29]

Pedestrian accidents occur to all age groups; however, a disproportionately large number of fatalities involve senior citizens and children. Approximately half of all pedestrian fatalities occur to these population groups. It may be that older individuals cannot cope with motor vehicle traffic as effectively as can younger adults because of certain physical impairments. Hearing loss makes it difficult to detect an oncoming car. Slowing of physical reactions may prevent the older pedestrian from getting out of the way of a fast-moving motor vehicle. Failing eyesight often becomes a hindrance for the elderly, especially problems with depth perception.

Children also are vulnerable because of their play activity that can take them into the pathway of moving vehicles. Pedestrian accidents rank second among the causes of death and injury for young children. Children need to receive instruction from their earliest years in safety behaviors that can help to reduce the possibility of pedestrian accidents among this population group.

Among the preschool population under five years of age, an all too common occurrence is the tendency for motorists to back over the child in the home driveway. This results from children playing near the vehicle. The operator of any motor vehicle must be extremely careful before backing up near locations where children are present.

Among five- to nine-year-old children, more than half of pedestrian accidents are mid-block dash or dart-out and intersection dash occurrences. Children have a tendency to look where they are going, not for oncoming vehicles. They look for a path between parked cars, not noting the oncoming traffic.

A common message often given to children about entering a street is "don't cross between parked cars." The effectiveness of this message is somewhat questionable.[30] A more successful recommendation is for the child to "look left, right, and left again to see if a car is coming." This encourages two looks aimed in the direction of the most immediate threat. It also discourages the likelihood of quick street entry. Education efforts targeting young school-age children should focus on preventing quick street entry and encouraging a deliberate search of the situation before entering the street.[31]

Pedestrian accidents occur because either the driver fails to see the individual or the pedestrian fails to see the approaching vehicle. No pedestrian should ever enter a roadway unless there is a clear field of vision. Pedestrians must walk on a sidewalk; if there is no sidewalk, they should walk facing the oncoming traffic. Wearing light-colored clothing or reflectorized garments helps visibility.

At night or at dusk, the individual on foot can easily blend into the surrounding darkness and not be noticed by the driver until it is too late. Any person walking, playing, or jogging along a roadway at dusk or after dusk should be expected to wear highly visible clothing or specific markings that are easily recognized. Retro-reflective materials, such as on vests or sashes, are particularly effective. When an individual is walking along a roadway after dark, a flashlight also can help improve visibility.

One of the greatest dangers in urban localities is the practice of crossing a street between intersections—jaywalking. In some cities a person can be fined for jaywalking. The wisest policy is to prohibit this action; however, this may not be feasible. Perhaps we would do well to teach people how to cross in the middle of the block safely rather than work to re-educate people to the dangers of jaywalking.

Safety at Rail Crossings

Special emphasis should be placed upon improving the many railroad crossings in the nation. Approximately 600 fatalities a year occur as the result of train and motor vehicle collisions. Railroad crossings must be clearly marked with warning flashers and gates. Also they need to be kept in safe repair so as to provide a smooth crossing for all motor vehicles.

Several causes for accidents at rail crossings have been identified. Many times the driver fails to obey warning signals and proceeds across a railroad track, intending to get across before the oncoming train arrives at the crossing. Misjudgment of the train's speed and distance is a contributing factor. Some rail crossing collisions have been reported in which the occupants of the motor vehicle were unable to hear the train whistle because of noise generated by a radio, air conditioner, or other occupants in the vehicle.

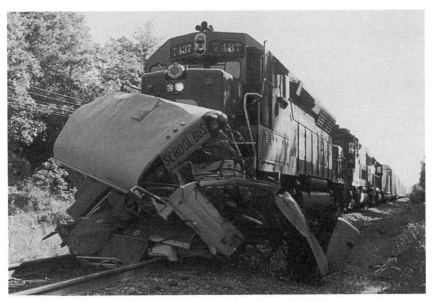

People riding in a motor vehicle have little chance when struck by a moving railroad engine. Special precautions should always be taken when crossing a railroad track.

Many rail collisions occur in rural localities where there is inadequate warning—i.e., usually the only warning signal is a sign that indicates there is a railroad crossing. There are no lighted signals or cross-bars. Crossing signals may be covered by surrounding shrubs, weeds, or trees; they may not be visible at dusk or after dark. Obviously, measures must be taken to eliminate as many of these types of crossing signs as possible.

Prevention of rail accidents should include the practice of watching the second track. One should not proceed just as the caboose or last railroad car passes since another train may be approaching on the second track. It is important to ensure good visibility of both tracks before proceeding to cross.

Summary

The development of motor vehicles has revolutionized life for many people throughout the world. The basic economic structure of most countries in the world is strongly affected by the financial condition of the automotive industry. As with many inventions and industrial developments, the value of the motor vehicle must be tempered by the fact that many fatalities and injuries occur daily resulting from vehicle use. In addition to the fatalities and injuries, the economic costs of motor vehicle collisions run into the billions of dollars.

A number of causes of motor vehicle crashes have been identified. Most involve a combination of factors—human, vehicular, and environmental in nature.

A major contributor to motor vehicle crashes is the combination of driving and use of alcoholic beverages. Nearly half of all fatal motor vehicle crashes involve drunk drivers. Numerous measures have been put in place to counter the problems associated with drunk driving. These include passage of implied consent laws, raising the legal drinking age, institution of dram shop laws, and various actions taken by law enforcement and consumer groups.

It is probably inevitable that motor vehicles will be involved to various degrees in collisions. The second collision—occurring instantly after the initial collision—results in the occupants being thrown about inside and/or out of the vehicle, and produces serious injuries and fatalities.

Various restraint systems have been manufactured designed to keep the occupant from being thrown about the vehicle. Active restraints—lap and shoulder belts—have been installed in most automobiles for several years. Legislation in a majority of states now requires the use of seat belts. Child restraint seats also are required in all states. In addition, passive restraints, particularly airbags, are now being included as part of the standard equipment of motor vehicles.

In recent years, speed limits have been increased from 55 to 65 miles per hour on rural interstate highways. This has resulted in increased driving speeds and higher related accident rates in most parts of the country.

Not only are individuals killed and injured while riding in motor vehicles, but many people are struck while walking or standing along a roadway. Measures can be taken to reduce the possibility of such pedestrian crashes.

Discussion Questions

1. Discuss the impact of the motor vehicle on society since its introduction in the early twentieth century.
2. What population groups are particularly at risk for fatality and injury from motor vehicles as identified in the national health objectives initiative for the year 2000?
3. Identify and be able to discuss the motor vehicle health objectives to be achieved by the year 2000.

4. Do you agree that the primary cause of motor vehicle crashes relates to human factors? Explain your answer.
5. Why do young people seem to have a disproportionately high percentage of automobile fatalities and injuries?
6. Explain the physiological effect of alcohol in the human body.
7. In what ways does alcohol use impede the operation of a motor vehicle?
8. What is meant by BAC?
9. What are implied consent laws?
10. Discuss the impact of the Uniform Minimum Drinking Age Law on the drinking and driving patterns of young people.
11. Explain how dram shop laws impact the issue of driving and drinking.
12. Discuss some of the recommendations of the Surgeon General's Workshop on Drunk Driving.
13. What is meant by first and second collision?
14. Do you support the mandated wearing of seat belts in all motor vehicles? Defend your answer.
15. What are some reasons given by people in opposition to airbags?
16. Do you support the raising of the speed limit to 65 miles per hour? Defend your answer.
17. Discuss several factors related to pedestrian safety.
18. Why do people have a tendency not to stop at railroad crossings when trains are approaching?

Suggested Readings

Asalor, J. O., and others. "Pure Circumstance in Road Traffic Accidents," *Journal of Safety Research* 25, no. 1 (Spring 1994): 47–60.

Baum, Herbert M., Jo Ann K. Wells, and Adrian K. Lund. "Motor Vehicle Crash Fatalities in the Second Year of 65 M.P.H. Speed Limits," *Journal of Safety Research,* 21 no. 1 (Spring 1990): 1–8.

Baum, Herbert M., and others. "The Fatality Consequences of the 65 mph Speed Limits, 1989," *Journal of Safety Research* 22, no. 4 (Winter 1991): 171–77.

Brison, Robert J., and others. "Fatal Pedestrian Injuries to Young Children: A Different Pattern of Injury," *American Journal of Public Health* 78, no. 7 (July 1988): 793–95.

Centers for Disease Control. "Alcohol-Related Traffic Fatalities—United States, 1982–1989," *Morbidity and Mortality Weekly Report* 39, no. 49 (14 December 1990): 889–91.

———. "Motor-Vehicle-Related Deaths Involving Intoxicated Pedestrians—United States, 1982–1992," *Morbidity and Mortality Weekly Report* 43, no. 14 (15 April 1994): 249–53.

Chang, Gang-Len, and others. "Intervention Analysis for the Impacts of the 65 mph Speed Limit on Rural Interstate Highway Fatalities," *Journal of Safety Research* 34, no. 1 (Spring 1993): 33–53.

"Child Safety Seats." *Consumer Reports* 57, no. 1 (January 1992): 16–20.

Colquitt, Mark, L. Peter Fielding, and John F. Cronan. "Drunk Drivers and Medical and Social Injury," *New England Journal of Medicine* 317, no. 20 (12 November 1987): 1262–66.

Feuerstein, Phyllis. "Rear Safety Belts Deserve Front Seat Attention," *Safety and Health* 145, no. 31 (March 1992): 64–65.

Gallagher, Margaret M., and others. "Effects of the 65 M.P.H. Speed Limit on Rural Interstate Fatalities in New Mexico," *Journal of the American Medical Association* 262, no. 16 (27 October 1989): 2243–45.

Hansotia, Phiroze, and Steven K. Broste. "The Effect of Epilepsy or Diabetes Mellitus on the Risk of Automobile Accidents," *The New England Journal of Medicine* 324, no. 1 (3 January 1991): 22–26.

Henderson, Al, and Catherine Kedjidjian. "New Laws Force Drunks Off the Road," *Safety and Health* 147, no. 3 (March 1993): 68–71.

Hingson, Ralph, and others. "Repeal of the Massachusetts Seat Belt Law," *American Journal of Public Health* 78, no. 5 (May 1988): 548–52.

Jones, Nancy E., and others. "The Effect of Legal Drinking Age on Fatal Injuries of Adolescents and Young Adults," *American Journal of Public Health* 82, no. 1 (January 1992): 112–14.

Latimer, Eric A., and Lester B. Lave. "Initial Effects of the New York State Auto Safety Belt Law," *American Journal of Public Health* 77, no. 2 (February 1987): 183–86.

Leary, Barbara F. "Court-Ordered Emergency Visitations for DUI Offenders," *The Journal of Emergency Medicine* 9, no. 1 (January–February 1991): 15–19.

Martin, Gary L., and Ian M. Newman. "Women as Motivators in the Uses of Safety Belts," *Health Values* 14, no. 6 (November–December 1990): 37–47.

Mortimer, R. G., and others. "Effects of Incentives and Enforcement on the Use of Seat Belts by Drivers," *Journal of Safety Research* 21, no. 1 (Spring 1990): 25–37.

Robertson, Leon B. "How to Save Fuel and Reduce Injuries in Automobiles," *The Journal of Trauma* 31, no. 1 (January 1991): 107–109.

Roth, Gabriel. "How to Improve America's Highways," *Consumers' Research* 74, no. 2 (February 1991): 11–15, 40.

Spencer, Peter L. "The Trouble With Airbags," *Consumers' Research* 74, no. 1 (January 1991): 10–13.

Stevenson, Mark R. "Analytical Approach to the Investigation of Childhood Pedestrian Injuries: A Review of the Literature," *Journal of Safety Research* 22, no. 3 (Fall 1991): 123–32.

Williams, Allan F., and others. "Use of Seatbelts in Cars With Automatic Belts," *Public Health Reports* 107, no. 2 (March–April 1992): 182–88.

Endnotes

1. Data reported in this chapter unless otherwise noted are from National Safety Council, *Accident Facts, 1993 Edition* (Itasca, IL: National Safety Council 1993), 54.
2. "First Auto Crash Victim Died 72 Years Ago Today," *Journal of the American Medical Association* 217, no. 11 (13 September 1971): 1461.
3. National Safety Council, *Accident Facts 1993,* 54.
4. Department of Health and Human Services, *Healthy People 2000: National Health Promotion and Disease Prevention Objectives* (Washington, DC: U.S. Government Printing Office, 1991), 274–75.
5. Gabriel Roth, "How to Improve America's Highways." *Consumers' Research* 74, no. 2 (February 1991): 11–15.
6. Department of Health and Human Services, *Healthy People 2000,* 166.
7. National Institute on Alcohol Abuse and Alcoholism, "Facts and Findings About Drinking and Driving," *Alcohol Health and Research World* 7, no. 1 (Fall 1982): 3.

8. Barbara F. Leary, "Court-Ordered Emergency Visitations for DUI Offenders," *The Journal of Emergency Medicine* 9 (1991): 19.
9. Ralph Hingson and others, "Effects of Legislative Reform to Reduce Drunken Driving and Alcohol-Related Traffic Fatalities," *Public Health Reports* 103, no. 6 (November–December 1988): 660.
10. Saeed Maghsoodloo, David B. Broan, and Perry A. Greathouse, "Impact of the Revision of DUI Legislation in Alabama," *American Journal of Drug and Alcohol Abuse* 14, no. 1 (1988): 97–108.
11. Michigan Drinking Legislation (1992).
12. Al Henderson and Catherine Kedjidjian, "New Laws Force Drunks Off the Road," *Safety and Health* 147, no. 3 (March 1993): 68–71.
13. Ibid.
14. Frederick L. McGuire, "The Accuracy of Estimating the Sobriety of Drinking Drivers," *Journal of Safety Research* 17, no. 2 (Summer 1986): 81–85.
15. Alan Hoskin and others, "The Effect of Raising the Legal Minimum Drinking Age on Fatal Crashes in 10 States," *Journal of Safety Research* 17, no. 3 (Fall 1986): 117–28.
16. Alexander C. Wagenear and Margaret B. T. Wiviott, "Effects of Mandating Seatbelt Use: A Series of Surveys on Compliance in Michigan," *Public Health Reports* 101, no. 5 (September–October 1986): 505–13.
17. Department of Health and Human Services, *Surgeon General's Workshop on Drunk Driving: Proceedings* (Rockville, MD: Office of the Surgeon General, 1989).
18. C. L. Straith, "Guest Passenger Injuries," *Journal of the American Medical Association* 137 (1973): 348–51.
19. Federal National Traffic and Motor Vehicle Safety Act of 1966.
20. National Safety Council, *Accident Facts 1993,* 58.
21. Allan F. Williams and others, "Seat Belt Use Law Enforcement and Publicity in Elmira, New York: A Reminder Campaign," *American Journal of Public Health* 77, no. 11 (November 1987): 1450–51.
22. Public information report issued by the National Highway Traffic Safety Administration, 1993.
23. Department of Health and Human Services, *Healthy People 2000,* 10–11.
24. "Child Safety Seats," *Consumer Reports* 57, no. 1 (January 1992): 16–20.
25. Ibid.

26. Peter L. Spencer, "The Trouble With Airbags," *Consumers' Research* 74, no. 1 (January 1991): 10–13.
27. Ibid.
28. National Safety Council, *Accident Facts 1993,* 58.
29. Ibid.
30. Kathryn E. H. Race, "Evaluating Pedestrian Safety Education Materials for Children Ages Five to Nine," *Journal of School Health* 58, no. 7 (September 1988): 277–81.
31. Ibid., 278.

CHAPTER 8

Forces of Nature—Cause of Many Fatalities and Injuries

Chapter Outline

Introduction
Tornadoes
Hurricanes
Lightning
Blizzards
Floods

Earthquakes
Summary
Discussion Questions
Suggested Readings
Endnotes

Introduction

Various forces of nature cause hundreds of thousands of fatalities, injuries, and extensive property damage each year throughout the world. In the United States some such catastrophic occurrence seems to take place each year. Sometimes more than one receives national attention. In addition individual, isolated events happen almost daily in some part of the country.

In some instances advanced planning may help to reduce fatalities, injuries, and property damage. More than likely, however, the natural calamity takes place with little advanced warning. Panic, fear, and secondary damage accompanying the event often cause as much chaos and injury as does the actual disaster.

Damage, destruction, and upheaval resulting from natural causes will continue as long as life exists on earth. Humans must learn to cope with the various forces of nature. There is need to develop earlier warning systems where possible. People must learn to take cover when there is danger of an approaching storm or cataclysm such as a tornado or a hurricane. They must heed warnings to evacuate their homes and other areas when conditions point to an impending potentially damaging natural event. Improved engineering and construction of public buildings, homes, schools, and other structures can provide protection for individuals when faced with a dangerous force of nature.

In any kind of natural disaster, community planning is essential. The role and responsibilities of law enforcement, fire, health, and safety agencies should be analyzed and identified as part of a coordinated community disaster preparedness program. The public must become better informed and educated about measures that can be taken to reduce the likelihood of death and injury occurring at the time of a natural disaster.

Disaster preparedness programs should include clear and comprehensive plans spelling out the actions to be taken throughout the community. Facilities for housing people who have been forced from their homes should be noted. The plan should identify measures that will need to be taken to provide for the medical needs. Agencies providing social services need to develop greater understanding of the emotional and psychological effects of exposure to violence caused by natural occurrences. Not only are relief services necessary at the time of the natural disaster, but long-term assistance to survivors is often necessary. These services include rehabilitation activities—physical, social, and psychological.

In the United States the majority of fatalities, personal injuries, and economic destruction caused by forces of nature can be attributed to tornadoes, lightning, blizzards, floods, earthquakes, and hurricanes.

Tornadoes

Tornadoes are one of the most lethal and violent atmospheric forces of nature. They have been known to occur throughout the United States. Most commonly they occur in the Midwest, the South, and in the Great Plains states.

Tornadoes strike suddenly and unpredictably. A *tornado,* also known as a twister, is a whirlwind formed along a front of warm, moist air and cool, dry air—usually developing during warm, humid, unsettled weather conditions. The effect is very high winds, sometimes reaching 100 to 300 miles per hour, and a sudden drop in air pressure at the storm's vortex. This air pressure drop causes an acceleration of wind speed. Rotation of the winds proceeds in a counterclockwise direction in the Northern Hemisphere; rotation is clockwise in the Southern Hemisphere.

The visual evidence of a tornado is the funnel cloud, extending downward from overhead thunderstorm clouds. That funnel is made up of fine waterdrops that condense in the region of low pressure and under the temperature that exists at the tornado's core. Windspeeds within the whirlpool often reach 300 or more miles per hour, with some recorded instances exceeding 500 miles per hour. The forward speed of the whole tornado averages 30 miles per hour, but can reach speeds of as much as 60 miles per hour. Normally tornadoes traverse from the southwest toward the northeast.

A tornado usually follows an unpredictable narrow path. The funnel may destroy everything in its pathway where it touches the ground. The powerful updraft of the wind patterns pulls up trees and can lift heavy objects. A tornado may strike one building and not touch the next; it may destroy a solid brick building, but not damage a wooden shed. A railroad engine may be blown some distance while a child's bicycle is left untouched.

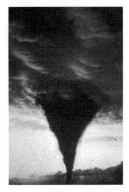

Tornadoes are funnel clouds that originate from overhead thunderstorm clouds. They usually follow unpredictable, narrow paths.

Tornadoes can occur at any time of the year when the weather conditions are right for their development. However, the months of April through July produce most twisters. Though they can occur at any time during the night or day, most occur between three and seven in the afternoon, at the maximum atmospheric heating time of the day. It is estimated that as many as 700 tornadoes occur each year in the United States.[1]

All ages are affected by tornadoes, but the elderly are particularly at risk for injury. This is because senior citizens tend to be less mobile and cannot escape to a place of protection and safety as readily as younger people. The elderly also may be less able to comprehend and react to tornado warnings.

Injuries from tornadoes may occur from the direct impact of the twister or from exposure to related conditions. Most impact-related injuries and fatalities occur instantaneously. Those that occur later are usually the result of complications after the initial impact. For instance, individuals may experience injury from falling debris. Also, injuries may result to those who are engaged in the clean-up operation in the aftermath of a tornado.

Numerous precautions can be taken to protect against an approaching tornado. Every family should plan and discuss appropriate measures to deal with such an emergency. Children should know where they are to go—to the basement, in closets, under furniture, or other designated safe locations in the house. Individuals living in apartments, university dormitories, or other high-rise housing units must be aware of the most appropriate places to go in case of a tornado. There should be a flashlight and portable radio available in case electricity is cut off, so that people can move to safety in the dark and can remain in contact with emergency weather reports on the radio.

The most important community-wide measure is informing the public of the possibility of an approaching tornado. Two kinds of tornado alerts have been designed to inform the public: a *tornado watch* and a *tornado warning*.

If the atmospheric conditions are ideal for the formation of a tornado, a *tornado watch* is issued. This does not mean that a tornado has been sighted. It only indicates that the public must be alerted because weather conditions could lead to development of a tornado. During a tornado watch one should remain informed by listening to the radio or television for further developments, warnings, and instructions.

A *tornado warning* is issued when a tornado has been sighted. If a warning is sounded, it is important to seek safe shelter immediately. This is not the time to go outdoors "looking" for the funnel. Time may be very important with just seconds available to find protection. Prearranged action should now be taken to ensure safety.

If a person is inside a building, particularly a house, it is best to go to the basement and remain until the danger has passed. In homes that have no basement, shelter should be taken in the center of the house. Closets or bathrooms without windows often serve as a protection. Shelter may be taken under heavy furniture or along the inside walls of rooms with windows and doors. Covering oneself with blankets and similar materials can provide limited protection from flying objects.

Though it was once believed and taught that people were safest in the southwest corners of a house or building, research following tornado strikes has indicated this to be an inaccurate concept. All too often the outside walls that are struck initially by the oncoming tornado fall on those in the southwest corner. There tends to be more protection in the center of the structure where the falling walls are not as likely to collapse on the occupants. Also, it is unnecessary to open windows with the oncoming approach of a tornado. Such action does not protect against inward collapse of the structure as was taught in the past.

People in mobile homes are particularly vulnerable to danger from the winds of a tornado. Such homes can be thrown about for great distances by the winds. Mobile homes also offer little structural support that can protect against outside objects falling on the structure. Obviously there are no basements to which occupants can escape for protection.

It is of little use to attempt to provide protection by tying down a mobile home. Tie downs, though they may provide some stability in normal conditions, provide virtually no protection at the time of a tornado strike. In the case of an approaching tornado and associated tornado warning, if at all possible, the mobile home should be abandoned, and the occupants should go to the nearest sturdy building. Any person residing in a mobile home should make emergency plans prior to a tornado warning. If there is no sturdy structure nearby, it is safer to go outside and lie in a ditch or ravine than to stay inside the trailer.

If an individual is caught outside with an approaching tornado, it is best to lie face down in the nearest land depression. A ravine or a ditch may provide a degree of protection. No attempt should be made to outrun or escape the tornado in a motor vehicle. In most cases this is impossible, and severe injury can occur should the motor vehicle be caught in the winds of the twister.

Every school should have a prearranged and practiced tornado warning drill. In many states schools are required to practice tornado drills as a part of the school emergency preparedness program. Generally it is advised that children go into a hall area and sit facing the wall. If it is necessary for them to remain in the classroom, the best procedure is to have the students get under their desks and cover their heads with their arms and hands to protect against any possible flying glass or other objects.

After the passage of a tornado, various actions will need to be taken by community agencies to make sure everyone affected is safe. Obviously a major responsibility at this time is to provide care to people with injuries and to protect against further injury. Particular care must be taken to protect against coming into contact with downed power lines.

If there has been a lot of damage in the area it will be important that law enforcement agencies become involved. Outsiders may need to be kept out of the affected area to protect against looting. Even the home owners may need to be kept out of the area until dangerous conditions associated with downed power lines, leaning or weakened structures, and other potential hazards can be eliminated.

Hurricanes

A *hurricane* is a whirlwind of air that moves in a large spiral. This air mass surrounds what is termed the "eye" of the hurricane, a relatively calm center of low barometric pressure within the whirlwind, with a diameter of up to 25 miles. Winds gusting from 75 miles per hour up to as much as 200 miles per hour surround the eye of the storm system. In order for a storm to be classified as a hurricane, winds of 75 miles per hour or higher must be maintained.

Hurricanes usually form over tropical oceans and, over a period of time, they begin to move in a northwesterly direction. As the hurricane moves over water, it increases in speed, size, and intensity. When the storm arrives over a landfall region, it tends to lose force; eventually it becomes downgraded to a heavy rainstorm.

The path that a hurricane is likely to take can be plotted fairly accurately. This does not guarantee that changes in direction will always be known in advance. However, general directional patterns can be predicted, and early warning given about landfall areas that are in danger.

The forward motion of a hurricane may be relatively slow, or the storm may remain stationary for certain periods of time. Forward motion is usually accelerated as a hurricane moves farther from the tropics and until it reaches landfall.

In the United States hurricanes principally have tended to affect the states along the Gulf of Mexico and along the eastern seaboard. The same natural phenomenon occurs in the Pacific Ocean. In the western Pacific and Indian oceans these phenomena are referred to as typhoons.

Because of improved weather forecasting and computer technology, it is increasingly possible to chart the progress of most hurricanes accurately. With only a small degree of error, weather forecasters can inform communities along the coastlines of the approach of a hurricane. Today communities and individuals often have adequate warning time in which to take precautions that protect property and people from danger. Steps need to be taken to board up buildings in the path of the approaching storm. Objects that might be blown about by the high winds need to be tied down. People must be encouraged to seek shelter in appropriate facilities.

The winds of a hurricane can cause damage and injury by uprooting trees and blowing down power lines. Torrential rains that usually accompany a hurricane produce heavy flooding, thus creating dangers associated with drowning, electrocution, and structural destruction.

In September 1989 Hurricane Hugo moved across parts of the Caribbean causing extensive damage to the Virgin Islands, Puerto Rico, and finally striking land near Charleston, South Carolina. Winds of this hurricane were recorded as high as 135 miles per hour. Heavy rains accompanied by tidal surges as high as 15 feet caused much damage, personal injury, and death.

Over 70 individuals were reported to have been killed from this hurricane throughout the Caribbean region to the South Carolina coast. About one-third of the fatalities were the direct result of the impact of

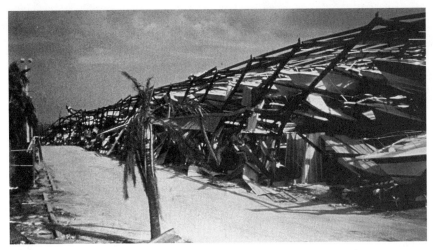

Hurricane Andrew caused mass destruction in southern Florida in 1992.

the hurricane; the other two-thirds resulted from postimpact conditions. These included fatalities from drownings, fires caused by the violence of the storm, and electrocutions.

Within a one-month period of time in August 1992, two of the most destructive hurricanes in history struck the United States: Hurricane Andrew in south Florida and Hurricane Iniki in Hawaii. Both of these hurricanes had winds in excess of 165 miles per hour. It is believed that the winds of Hurricane Andrew may have reached 200 miles per hour. It is uncertain exactly how high these winds became because the wind-speed measurement technology of the National Weather Center in Florida was "knocked out" due to the close proximity to the storm. Hurricane Andrew moved forward at a speed of about 20 miles per hour, about twice the normal rate of forward movement of such a hurricane.[2] Eventually it reached landfall a second time in Louisiana.

South Florida was particularly hard hit. An estimated $30 billion of damage was recorded. Whole communities were destroyed, particularly the city of Homestead, Florida. Some 250,000 people were left homeless, and thousands were left without jobs. Though the numbers of people affected and economic loss caused by Hurricane Andrew in Louisiana and Hurricane Iniki in Hawaii was not as great, the total destruction was as great as in Florida.

If there was any positive factor in these particular natural disasters it was that only 14 people died as a direct result of Hurricane Andrew. Another 20 or more died from storm-related causes. For example, there were a number of reported fatalities due to heart attacks. A major reason given for this relatively low number of fatalities was the fact that residents heard the National Weather Service warnings for several days and left the area.

Many of the injuries that occurred in conjunction with these hurricanes involved circumstances following the passage of the strong winds and rains. The public also must be made aware of the risks of injuries during clean-up operations, particularly from hazards relating to power outages, downed electrical wires, and fires. In addition, there were many health and basic social problems that resulted. In south Florida there were food and water shortages. With electrical power out, there was no refrigeration in many localities for days—causing spoilage of refrigerated foodstuffs. Also, transportation became nearly impossible. Thousands of cars were destroyed; roads were totally blocked making travel even related to necessary services a most difficult matter for some time.

It is important that communities and individuals located in the pathway of an approaching hurricane recognize the importance of evacuation from the area. In the case of Hurricanes Hugo, Andrew, and Iniki, various community health, safety, and social agencies were involved in providing services during the early warning period and in the coordination of evacuation efforts. Obviously law enforcement personnel play important roles in the evacuation process. People must be adequately informed of the potential danger and be required to leave when necessary. Following the passage of the hurricanes, these various agencies provided numerous emergency care services.

As with tornadoes, hurricanes are of particular risk for those individuals living in mobile homes. In southern Florida, Hurricane Andrew completely obliterated a number of mobile home parks. Study of such structures hit by Hurricane Andrew have revealed that mobile homes tended to blow apart.[3] As they disintegrated, parts were thrown about like shrapnel. This presented tremendous potential for human injury.

Evacuation must be a part of any community emergency preparedness plan. Available community facilities must be identified where all citizens can go for protection. Moreover, routes and procedures for evacuation must be developed for individuals living on coastal islands and peninsulas. This has been a particularly important issue along the Outer Banks of the Carolina coast where there is only one roadway off the islands. Such emergencies are not the time for major highway congestion and traffic control conflicts.

Study of the damage done by Hurricane Andrew in Florida has shown the importance of enforcing hurricane prevention building codes and regulations. In localities where such storms are a potential hazard, all buildings must have hurricane-proof construction. Shutters should be available for windows to protect the glass from shattering. In Florida following Hurricane Andrew, a controversy arose as to whether community building codes had been adequate and had been enforced. Many homes had been built with stapled roof shingles, and wallboard had been used for wall sidings. Though these structures were supposed to withstand winds of up to 120 miles per hour, many experts doubt whether these homes could have survived with winds of that speed. It continues to be important that construction engineers develop more effective buildings to withstand the high winds of hurricanes. Then building codes also must be established and enforced to provide protection for people living in parts of the country at high risk for hurricanes.

Lightning

Although not classified as a natural calamity, lightning is a natural phenomenon that causes the death of nearly a hundred people annually.[4] Deaths often result from injuries and brain damage associated with the flow of electricity as it passes through the human body. The majority of these fatalities occur on golf courses, at the beach, or on baseball/softball diamonds. Two-thirds of the victims of lightning strikes are not killed instantly.[5] In most instances these individuals are in need of immediate emergency rescue activities.

There are many people who are struck by lightning who are not killed but who experience a variety of serious injuries. For example, burns are often noted on areas of the body near a metal object such as a zipper, keys, or a chain. Wearing polyester clothes can contribute to serious injuries because this type of clothing sometimes is melted by the flow of electricity from the lightning. The result can be extensive third-degree burns.

Lightning is a discharge of electricity that begins in a thundercloud. As the thundercloud passes overhead, two opposite-charged bodies—the cloud and the earth's surface—come into proximity and a bolt of electricity passes from the cloud through the air toward the ground.

Any object that protrudes upward from the earth's surface and is a conductor of electricity may "attract" the bolt of lightning. Trees, television towers, telephone poles, and church steeples may be at risk. A person moving across an open area such as a farm field, a lake, or a golf course is subject to being struck by a bolt of lightning.

LIGHTNING STRIKE PREVENTIVE MEASURES

1. Get inside a house or other large building or inside a vehicle when there is the likelihood of lightning occurring.
2. Do not use the telephone or come into close contact with plugged electrical appliances when it is lightning.
3. Do not stand under tall, isolated trees.
4. Do not project above the surrounding landscape.
5. Stay away from open water.
6. Stay away from any metal farm equipment.
7. Stay away from bicycles, motorcycles, and golf carts in the presence of lightning.
8. Put golf clubs down when it is lightning.
9. Stay away from metallic objects that can serve as a path for lightning, such as drain pipes and antennas.
10. Do not stand in small, isolated sheds.
11. Seek shelter in a low area under a thick growth of small trees.
12. In open areas, go into a valley or a ravine.

Source: United States National Weather Service, general information publications.

Any type of outdoor activity when the atmospheric conditions are appropriate for an electrical storm places an individual at risk. Agricultural and construction workers are in particular danger. It has been shown that fatalities occur not just with those who are directly struck by the bolt of lightning, but also with persons who are within 30 feet of where the lightning has hit.

When caught in a thunderstorm, do not seek shelter beside an object that rises alone above the landscape. Standing under a tree in a thunderstorm or holding an umbrella are potentially dangerous actions. Umbrellas, with their metal components, are good conductors of electrical current.

An individual should get off a beach or away from a body of water during a thunder-and-lightning storm. Water is a very attractive conductor of the electricity in the lightning.

On a golf course in a thunderstorm a person should move away from the golf clubs, as they can be conductors of electricity. When riding in a car in a thunderstorm, close all windows; lightning bolts have been known to pass through an open window. If caught out-of-doors in an electrical storm an individual should drop to the knees and bend forward with hands placed on the knees. Do not lie flat on the ground.

People need to become aware of how to protect themselves and others from the possibility of being struck by lightning. The United States Weather Service has prepared a series of important guidelines to know and follow.

Blizzards

Most states in the northern part of the United States are covered by snow during the winter months. People living in these areas learn to cope with various amounts of snow, ice, and cold weather conditions. One must pay particular attention when walking on slippery walks and roadways to protect against a fall that could result in injury. Driving a motor vehicle demands that one learn particular skills, both for operating the vehicle and braking on snow-covered roads. Communities in such regions usually have snow removal equipment available so that traffic is minimally impaired and life can continue at a normal pace.

People living in cold winter climates also learn to adapt to extremely cold temperatures by wearing appropriate clothing. Coping with snow, ice, and cold temperatures becomes a normal part of winter living. Wearing heavy winter jackets, protection for the head, the hands, and feet are all a normal consideration during this time of the year.

Periodically an area receives an abnormal amount of snow or the snowfall is accompanied by very high winds. These conditions are referred to as *blizzards*. According to the United States Weather Bureau, winds of 35 miles an hour or greater classify a snowstorm as a blizzard. During these conditions visibility is reduced and drifting snow makes travel nearly impossible. Such circumstances can be quite dangerous to anyone caught outside during the storm.

Blizzards can have a major impact upon business, commerce, and travel. When the airport in cities such as Denver, Minneapolis, or Chicago are closed for a number of hours due to blizzard conditions, travel patterns to other cities throughout the nation can be affected. Blizzards can prevent people from getting to school or to work. Individuals involved in service professions at hospitals and elsewhere often have to work extra hours to fill the roles of those who cannot get to work. Schools and shopping malls may be closed due to blizzard conditions.

In addition to the economic losses and disruption of everyday life, blizzards contribute to human injuries and fatalities. For instance, the winds and weight of the snow may cause downed power lines and curtail electrical services. The weight of the snow on trees and roofs of houses and other buildings may cause injury should they collapse.

Though storms of the magnitude of a blizzard are experienced regularly throughout the Snow Belt states and in Alaska, on occasion a particularly serious one occurs that is remembered for years afterward. During the winter of 1976–1977 the city of Buffalo, New York, a locality accustomed to heavy snowfalls in the winter, experienced a blizzard for five days, with snow and high winds that marooned thousands of motorists and paralyzed the city.

In March 1992 an unusual blizzard moved out of the southern states and struck north along the east coast causing widespread damage and bringing much of the Southeast and the eastern seaboard to a standstill. This snowstorm was particularly newsworthy since it affected parts of the country that never experience blizzards. Cities as far south as Birmingham, Alabama were affected. In the mountainous regions of the Carolinas and Virginia as much as four to five feet of snow fell. Since this storm occurred in the early spring, hundreds of thousands of motorists and individuals were stranded without proper warm clothing, gloves, and boots. Without shovels to help dig out stalled motor vehicles many people were stuck for hours.

One particular danger associated with blizzards is the threat of becoming stranded in a car along a roadway. When this occurs, the individual should elect to stay in the vehicle where it is possible to remain warm and safe from the elements. However, consideration must be given to the possible length of time that it may take for assistance to arrive. There is some question whether the engine should be kept running until help appears. For one thing, the amount of fuel available will help to decide if this measure is the best action to take. In addition, the danger of asphyxiation from carbon monoxide poisoning is great. When the motor is kept running, it is vital that the vehicle's tailpipe be kept free of snow and that a window or two be slightly open to protect against any build-up of carbon monoxide and to provide safe levels of oxygen.

Leaving the motor vehicle to seek assistance is a particularly dangerous action. With low temperatures and heavily blowing snow it is very easy for anyone walking to become lost and disoriented. An individual may think he or she knows where to go, but missing a road sign or other landmark by just a few feet is quite easy under the circumstances.

Because of the high blizzard winds, extremely low wind chill factors are often reported. *Wind chill* is the estimated temperature that is felt on the skin of a person. When wind comes into contact with human skin, the body temperature drops. Increased velocity of the wind can make the temperature a person experiences significantly lower than the reading on the thermometer. Such thermometer readings indicate only the temperature of the air without consideration of any wind movement.

In blizzard conditions exposure to wind chill factors of minus 40 degrees Fahrenheit or below are not unusual. For example, exposure to wind of 10 miles per hour with air temperature conditions of 20 degrees Fahrenheit results in a wind chill factor of about 2 degrees Fahrenheit. Thus, with winds of 35 miles per hour or greater and with air temperatures even in the twenties, the wind chill factor can be extremely dangerous—much below zero. Exposure to such extremely cold temperatures for only a few seconds or minutes can cause serious tissue damage, frostbite, hypothermia, and death.

It is wise for individuals living in regions where blizzards can occur to take a number of protective measures. One should always dress properly for cold winter weather. It also is important to carry certain emergency items in the vehicle to provide protection should one be caught in a storm. Extra warm jackets, blankets, boots, and gloves should be carried automatically in the car in the winter. A shovel is helpful should one be trapped in heavy snow. Old rugs, tire chains, sand, salt, and traction mats can be very useful when a vehicle is caught in snow. It is recommended that extra weight be carried in the trunk of a car—particularly smaller, lighter cars—during winter months. This added weight will help improve traction in the snow and on icy roadways.

Following a blizzard or any heavy snowstorm, many people remove the snow from their walks and driveways by shoveling or with the use of snowblowers. Without realizing the amount of energy output needed for such a task, they risk overexertion which could lead to a heart attack. It is important that an individual knows the safe limits within which he or she can work at the strenuous task of snow removal without causing harm to the cardiovascular system. One should lift only small amounts of snow at a time and should rest periodically. This will provide some protection against heart attack.

Floods

Worldwide, flooding is the most common natural disaster.[6] *Flooding* occurs when water rises to potentially hazardous levels, either rapidly or gradually. There may be a dam break in which a wall of water moves down a valley inundating land, towns, roadways, and people in a very short period of time. On the other hand, the flooding of a major river system, such as occurred in the Midwest in the summer of 1993, occurs

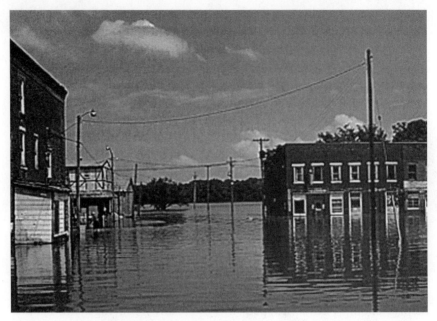

Flooding along the Mississippi River in 1993 resulted in much damage to communities for miles.

more gradually. Flooding may be the result of a large amount of rainfall or a snow melt when the ground cannot absorb all of the water.

In the United States floods occur in a variety of localities. It is estimated that about 200 fatalities occur in the United States from flooding each year.[7]

Some floods that take place in the United States are highly predictable. Communities in the path of the oncoming flood can take measures such as sandbagging buildings and homes to provide protection. It is not unusual during the spring of the year, as heavy snowmelt occurs along the upper regions of the Missouri and Mississippi rivers, for widespread flooding to occur. When a winter with a large accumulation of snow is followed by a rapid spring thaw or by heavy spring rains, flooding is to be expected.

This is what happened during the spring and summer of 1993. There was widespread flooding and much damage—both economically and in terms of livestock losses—in nine midwestern states. Extensive crop damage occurred on hundreds of farms. In Des Moines, Iowa the municipal water system was put out of operation for a period of time because of flooding. Homes were without tap water, water had to be trucked in, and people had to go to public facilities to get usable water.

It is the *flash flood*—precipitated by unusually heavy rainfall over a relatively short period of time—that causes the greatest amount of human injury and death. As the result of a sudden, heavy accumulation of water in a localized area, normal water tributaries overflow. When runoff systems overflow, water pours into areas from which it should be moving away. This type of flooding can catch a community by surprise, without adequate time to warn the citizens. Though flash floods can occur in many different localities, they tend to be particular risks in mountainous areas where quiet flowing streams and rivers suddenly become raging torrents as they move along narrow canyons.

There are other causes of dangerous flooding. Earthquakes often set into motion huge waves over large bodies of water, creating extensive damage and flooding on the shore some distance away from the quake epicenter. This results in what is known as a *tsunami*. Tsunamis caused major destruction in Hilo, Hawaii in 1946 and Alaska in 1964.

Flooding also can occur downstream from dams. Often following heavy rain the pressure of water in a lake behind a dam becomes so great that the dam gives way. Of particular concern are earthen dams that can become weakened by a lengthy period of rainfall and moisture buildup in the ground. In these circumstances flooding can occur with little warning to the surrounding population.

In order to reduce the likelihood of human injury and property damage associated with flooding, it is important that community planning measures be considered. People may need to be moved from low-lying regions along rivers and streams. One of the major questions that has been raised following the flooding in the Midwest in 1993 was how much settlement should be permitted on flood plains along the major rivers. Thousands of acres of farmland is cultivated on these flood plains located along rivers like the Mississippi. The more settlement and construction of houses and other buildings in these localities, the greater the possibility of economic damage and potential danger to human life.

In the case of an impending flood, farmers and other agricultural workers will need to make provisions for moving cattle and valuable farming equipment to higher ground. Cooperation and action by various community agencies will be required in order to minimize property damage and injury.

Earthquakes

Throughout human history, hundreds of thousands of people have lost their lives due to earthquakes. In possibly the greatest incidence of destruction from natural violence in recorded history, some 830,000 people in China were reported to have been killed in an earthquake in 1556.

More recently, in 1976 nearly a quarter of a million people were reported to have been killed in an earthquake in the interior of China. An earthquake in Mexico City in 1985 killed an estimated 30,000 individuals and left thousands homeless. In one hospital that was destroyed by the earthquake, several hundred patients, physicians, nurses, and other employees were killed.

For most Americans, except those living in the Pacific Coast states, a damaging earthquake is not a personal reality. It is something described in newspapers, magazines, or on television news broadcasts. The events of October 17, 1989 changed that sense of distance. As millions of Americans were settling into their chairs to watch the World Series from San Francisco, the announcer stated that an earthquake was in progress. For the next several hours those same millions of people who had planned to watch a baseball game saw live on television the devastating effects of yet another killer earthquake along the San Andreas Fault on the West Coast.

When the total damage from this earthquake was ascertained, more than 60 deaths were recorded, nearly 4,000 individuals suffered injuries necessitating emergency medical attention, and thousands of houses, apartments, and business establishments were damaged or destroyed. Nearly two-thirds of the deaths occurred when occupants of motor vehicles were trapped as the upper deck of a double-level freeway collapsed in Oakland, California. Tons of concrete came down on unsuspecting individuals who had no hope of escape.

The most devastating earthquake in United States history in terms of fatalities occurred in 1906 in San Francisco. Official data recorded that there were about 450 deaths. However, some historical researchers suggest that the true number of fatalities may have exceeded 3,000.[8]

Minor earth tremors are felt throughout much of the North American continent. However, the most destructive ones occur along the fault lines through California, Alaska, and the Rocky Mountain region. Several earthquakes registering six or more on the Richter scale occurred in California during 1992, further heightening fears of a coming "killer quake."

The *Richter scale* is a unit of measurement used to record and compare the strength of earthquakes. A Richter scale measurement of five or less is considered to be minor—i.e., likely to result in little serious damage. A reading of seven or more indicates an earthquake that has potential for causing much injury, death, and property damage.

An *earthquake* is the result of great pressures brought about as slabs of the earth's crust rub against each other. These pressures are exerted as the earth moves ever so slightly. When these pressures

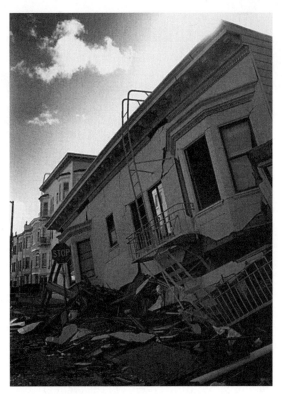

Earthquake damage in San Francisco, 1989.

become greater than the rock layers can endure, a snapping and shifting movement results. The movement of the ground during a quake is measured by a seismograph.

Scientific research has improved the predictability of possible earthquakes. Several systems are used to predict the onset of an earthquake, such as counting the microquakes and recording their buildup over a period of time. By means of laser beam, light-wave movement in the earth's crust of as little as twenty trillionths of an inch can be recorded.[9]

Alarm systems have been developed in parts of the country where earthquakes are most likely to occur to notify people that conditions are present for such an emergency. These early earthquake warning procedures are useful. Yet, in order for them to be most effective, they must be accurate. False announcements will lead people to ignore legitimate attempts at early earthquake warning.

It is doubtful if measures can be developed to protect everyone from the destruction accompanying major quakes. However, it is important to know and practice effective measures for the protection of

Forces of Nature—Cause of Many Fatalities and Injuries

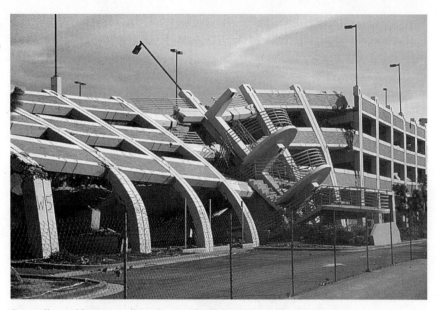

Regardless of how "earthquake proof" buildings are thought to be constructed, damage can still occur resulting from a major earthquake as occurred in Los Angeles in early 1994.

citizens. Increasingly, building codes in areas that are earthquake prone have taken into consideration the need for constructing earthquake-proof facilities. Homes and office buildings can be designed and constructed to prevent building collapse during an earthquake. For example, steel reinforced concrete slabs under buildings provide a foundation that can absorb the shocks of an earthquake. The use of anchor bolts helps to secure the building to this foundation.[10] Buildings constructed of structural steel and reinforced concrete tend to withstand earthquakes quite well. The value of constructing buildings with earthquake protection in mind was demonstrated in the 1989 San Francisco quake when the majority of modern structures in that area were not seriously damaged.

Another concern, in addition to collapsing structures, that must be considered during an earthquake is the matter of broken gas lines and water pipes. The gas leaking from broken lines can ignite and explode, causing extensive damage and triggering destructive fires. Fallen electrical wires also are a threat to those in the earthquake area, as is the case with other catastrophes involving forces of nature. Following an earthquake, water should be shut off if lines have been damaged or broken; the same applies to the main gas valve. Windows in a structure should be opened if there is any possibility of a gas line leak.

Although immediate efforts must concentrate on locating the injured and trapped and on rendering emergency aid, it is important to stay away from damaged structures because of the aftershocks that normally accompany a major earth tremor. These aftershocks, though usually of lesser strength than the original quake, may be strong enough to cause additional damage to already weakened structures. The result may be additional death and injury.

The importance of earthquake preparedness cannot be overemphasized. Most communities in earthquake prone regions have established emergency planning. The need to educate the public about appropriate measures that can, and should, be taken at the time of an earthquake has become a part of most community earthquake emergency planning programs. Community shelters have been identified where people can go for help, assistance, and safety. In many school districts along the West Coast, earthquake drills are practiced on a regular basis so that children will know how to protect themselves during a quake.

Summary

When mass disasters result from the forces of nature, many of the safety agencies within a community are called upon to meet the needs of the injured. Commonly, injuries and fatalities result from tornadoes, hurricanes, lightning, blizzards, floods, and earthquakes.

Tornadoes are very unpredictable, striking suddenly and causing much destruction along their paths. Early warning signals have been developed to inform the public of atmospheric conditions that are likely to result in a tornado. It is necessary to take swift preventive measures to protect oneself against the winds and accompanying destruction of a tornado.

Hurricanes are another natural force in which extremely high winds can lead to massive destruction. The movement of a hurricane is much more defined than that of a tornado. In recent years several hurricanes have hit different parts of the United States resulting in billions of dollars of property damage and numerous injuries. Fortunately, partially due to early warning and associated evacuation planning, fatalities have been at a minimum.

Lightning is the discharge of large amounts of electrical energy. Death and serious injuries can result from being struck by lightning. When caught out-of-doors with an approaching thunder-and-lightning storm, there are several precautions that protect against being struck by lightning.

Blizzards and flooding are other natural occurrences that can cause extensive damage, injury, as well as fatalities. Each needs to be understood, along with measures that can protect against them.

Earthquakes can cause the death and injury of thousands of people. Although they are not very predictable, certain strategies can prevent injury when one occurs. Building construction is one factor that can minimize damage, injury, and loss of life at the time of an earthquake. With an understanding of what can take place during and after an earthquake, individuals can take appropriate steps to protect themselves.

Discussion Questions

1. Discuss the forces of nature that result in a tornado.
2. Explain the difference between a hurricane and a tornado.
3. What is the difference between a tornado watch and a tornado warning?
4. What safety precautions must be taken under each tornado advisory condition—a tornado warning and a tornado watch?
5. When caught outside with a tornado approaching, what precautions should one take?
6. Discuss some of the impact of Hurricanes Hugo, Andrew, and Iniki.
7. What is lightning?
8. Identify several preventive measures that can protect an individual from being struck by lightning.
9. If stalled in a car during a blizzard, is it better to remain in the car or to leave the vehicle and walk to the nearest building for help? Discuss the reasons for the answer you have given.
10. What is the wind chill factor?
11. Discuss the different types of flooding with a focus on the specific dangers of each.
12. What were some of the factors associated with the flooding in the Midwest in the summer of 1993?
13. What is an earthquake?
14. Discuss some of the dangers related to earthquakes.

Suggested Readings

Canby, Thomas Y. "Earthquake: Prelude to the Big One?" *National Geographic* 177, no. 5 (May 1990): 76–105.

Centers for Disease Control. *Beyond the Flood: A Prevention Guide for Personal Health and Safety.* Atlanta, GA: Public Health Service, CDC (1993).

———. "Earthquake Disaster—Luzon, Philippines," *Morbidity and Mortality Weekly Report* 39, no. 34 (31 August 1990): 573–77.

———. "Preliminary Report: Medical Examiner Reports of Deaths Associated with Hurricane Andrew—Florida, August 1992," *Morbidity and Mortality Weekly Report* 41, no. 35 (4 September 1992): 641–44.

———. "Public Health Consequences of a Flood Disaster—Iowa, 1993." *Morbidity and Mortality Weekly Report* 42, no. 34 (3 September 1993): 653–55.

———. "Tornado Disaster—Alabama, March 27, 1994," *Morbidity and Mortality Weekly Report* 43, no. 19 (20 May 1994): 356–58.

Duclos, Philippe J., Lee M. Sanderson, and Karl C. Klontz. "Lightning—Related Mortality and Morbidity in Florida," *Public Health Reports* 105, no. 3 (May–June 1990): 276–82.

Gore, Rick. "Andrew Aftermath." *National Geographic* 183, no. 4 (April 1993): 1–37.

Lee, L. E., and others. "Active Morbidity Surveillance After Hurricane Andrew—Florida, 1992," *Journal of the American Medical Association* 270 (1993): 591–94.

Newcott, William R. "Lightning: Nature's High-Voltage Spectacle," *National Geographic* 184, no. 1 (July 1993): 83–103.

Endnotes

1. Centers for Disease Control, "Tornado Disaster—Illinois, 1990," *Morbidity and Mortality Weekly Report* 40, no. 2 (18 January 1991): 35.
2. Rick Gore, "Andrew Aftermath," *National Geographic* 183, no. 4 (April 1993): 18.

3. Ibid., 37.
4. William R. Newcott, "Lightning: Nature's High-Voltage Spectacle," *National Geographic* 184, no. 1 (July 1993): 90.
5. Philippe J. Duclos, Lee M. Sanderson, and Karl C. Klontz, "Lightning—Related Mortality and Morbidity in Florida," *Public Health Reports* 105, no. 3 (May–June 1990): 279.
6. Centers for Disease Control, "Health Consequences of a Flood Disaster—Iowa, 1993," *Morbidity and Mortality Weekly Report* 42, no. 34 (3 September 1993): 653.
7. Ibid.
8. Thomas Y. Canby, "Earthquake: Prelude to the Big One?" *National Geographic* 177, no. 5 (May 1990): 95.
9. Samuel W. Mathews, "This Changing Earth," *National Geographic* 143, no. 1 (January 1973): 31.
10. Ibid.

CHAPTER 9

Recreational Pursuits—Leisure Time Activities and the Need for Safety

Chapter Outline

Introduction
Motorized Recreational Vehicles
  Snowmobiles
  Motorcycles
  Minibikes
  All-Terrain Vehicles (ATVs)
Outdoor Recreational Activities
  Camping
  Hunting
  Skiing
Cycling
  The Bicycle—a Toy or Not?
  Cycle Construction and Operation
  Personal Gear
  Rules of the Road
Public Playgrounds
Summary
Discussion Questions
Suggested Readings
Endnotes

Introduction

Americans spend more time, energy, and money on recreational pursuits today than at any other time in history. Increasingly, individuals from all types of occupations and varying age groups are spending their leisure time participating in a wide range of recreational activities. Young families may use a weekend afternoon to go to a park so their children can enjoy the playground. People of all ages are involved in individual or group sporting activities. Many drive motorized recreational vehicles. For others, outdoor activities such as fishing, hiking, hunting, or camping are the source of recreation.

If projections are correct, leisure time and related recreational pursuits will increase in the years to come. This growing availability of leisure time is not limited to the young adult of college age or the employed segment of the American population. Elderly retired individuals are a rapidly growing population in the United States—a trend in part attributable to increased longevity. For a variety of reasons thousands of individuals also are taking early retirement. In some cases retirement is being forced on active people during their middle years because of corporate economic reductions. Other individuals choose to take early retirement in order to pursue different types of work and activities. Regardless of the factors that explain the increase in retired persons, most of these individuals have extended time for recreational pursuits. In short, opportunities for participation in recreational activities are likely to expand.

This focus on leisure necessitates the development of new interests and skills for many people. Skiing, swimming, cycling, and participation in individual sports such as golf, tennis, and racketball all involve skills that take time and effort to learn and to perfect. Hence, there is and will continue to be need for classes and instruction in the development of such recreational skills. These programs must be well taught; in turn, participants should be encouraged, and in some instances required by legislation, to attend.

It is especially important to learn appropriate safety rules and regulations. The use of individual equipment and high-powered machines, and exposure to unfamiliar environmental settings represent potential hazards that require planned instructional initiatives. For example, it is folly for a person to get behind the wheel of a snowmobile without first knowing something about the operation of the vehicle, its braking mechanism, and other related technical matters. Inexperienced hunters can cause problems for themselves, as well as for other hunters, if guns are not handled properly. Every recreational activity demands that participants exhibit sufficient individual physical conditioning to be able to function in a safe and healthful manner.

Recreation is becoming a year-round enterprise. In the past when cold weather, snow, and ice arrived, many people stayed indoors out of the elements and began planning for the next spring and summer. Some indoor activities were programmed, but little interest or thought was aimed at outdoor recreational pursuits during the winter months. Only the very young or hardy cold weather enthusiasts went skiing, ice skating, or ice fishing. However, in recent years increased interest in winter sport activities has emerged.

There are various categories of recreational pursuits. Some activities involve the use of motorized vehicles; others involve human mobility. Some recreational activities take place indoors, while others involve exposure to natural environments that require participants to function safely in outdoor settings.

Motorized Recreational Vehicles

Some types of recreational activities depend on the use of motor-driven vehicles. Whenever motorized vehicles are involved, the potential for serious injury and even death is always present. Individuals must be expected to handle such vehicles in a safe manner. There are certain basic principles that must be understood before a person should operate such a recreational vehicle.

Snowmobiles

The development and growth in popularity of the snowmobile has opened opportunities for thousands to experience the beauty of the out-of-doors in winter in many different locations throughout the United States. A *snowmobile* is a motorized vehicle which maneuvers on a pair of metal skis combined with a rubber belt tread. It is possible to travel by snowmobile over terrain previously inaccessible on foot in cold, snowy winter environments. The thrill of traveling through winter beauty—the serenity of a woods or a mountain valley isolated from roads and normal vehicular traffic—is part of the recreational appeal of the snowmobile. The mobility of this vehicle enables people to traverse large areas in relatively short periods of time.

Not only is the snowmobile an exciting recreational vehicle for use during one's leisure time, but it also performs a valuable service as an emergency vehicle in many locations. In times of severe winter storms when people otherwise have been stranded, the snowmobile can provide emergency supplies and rescue services. The vehicle is a common conveyance for many individuals in isolated communities of northern states and in parts of Canada.

In addition to these uses of the snowmobile, interest also has developed in snowmobile racing. In some localities snowmobile race tracks are kept busy through much of the winter. There are several major regional and national races that attract a diverse group of drivers, as well as spectators.

With the increasing numbers of snowmobiles, the probability of fatalities and injuries has also grown. Snowmobiles are able to travel at very high rates of speed; some can reach speeds of 80 to 100 miles

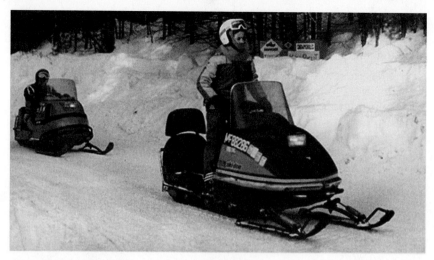

Care must be taken in the operation of a snowmobile.

per hour. Any movement at high rates of speed over terrain not designed for such movement presents the potential for a variety of different kinds of serious injuries.

A common cause of snowmobile collisions is driving at night at speeds that "overshoot" the lighting system of the vehicles. This means that the illumination provided by the vehicle lights does not extend far enough for the driver to bring the snowmobile to a halt before a collision results. Obviously, it is extremely important to operate snowmobiles after dark at speeds at which the vehicles can be kept under control.

The basic structure of snowmobiles and the nature of their operation mean that any collision is likely to result in serious injuries to the driver and riders. Snowmobiles have been known to collide with other snowmobiles, with motor vehicles on highways, with trains, trees, and other objects. The vehicles have run into deer in the woods of northern Minnesota and Wisconsin. Collisions of any kind while riding a snowmobile are dangerous because seat belt restraints are not included on most of these vehicles; an individual easily can be thrown from the vehicle upon impact.

One of the thrills of operating a snowmobile is being able to ride over terrain where no wheeled vehicle can go, including across frozen lakes and rivers. The very freedom felt in such settings presents possibilities for many different types of injury-causing situations. For example, before an individual drives out on ice, it is important to make sure that the surface is thick enough to hold the weight of the vehicle and its occupants.

Riding a snowmobile across a terrain of packed snow can result in significant jarring and bumping. Snowmobile riders must be advised to support their weight on their feet and ride the machine as if they were posting a horse. Neither the seat nor the vehicle itself absorbs the impact of bumps. Riding with one's weight supported by sitting on the seat may result in severe jolts that can cause serious back injuries. The most frequent injury from riding snowmobiles is a compression of the vertebrae in the thoracic and lumbar region of the back.

Not only do snowmobile collisions occur because of human error, but there may be mechanical failure as well. For example, failure of the braking system, damaged or broken skis, and jamming of throttle controls can all result in loss of control and associated serious injury. It is not unusual for the controls to become stuck or frozen, creating the potential for a serious collision.

The likelihood of being isolated miles from help with a damaged or incapacitated machine is a serious concern. At these times riders may be exposed to frostbite or other severe problems related to hypothermia. For this reason, no one should travel alone in rural or wilderness areas on snowmobiles.

It also is important that everyone riding a snowmobile be properly clothed. The rider of a snowmobile must take measures to keep warm at all times while outdoors. The cold natural temperature combined with the speed of movement of the vehicle may create wind chill factors of 50 degrees Fahrenheit or more below zero on the skin of the individual. In addition to warm clothing, all snowmobile riders should wear goggles and fastened helmets. Care must be taken to assure that the individual on a snowmobile does not have any loose clothing. Loose clothing, such as scarves might become caught on fences or overhanging tree limbs causing very serious injury.

With the increasing presence of snowmobiles, some states and local communities now prohibit their use in certain areas. Operation on public roads is limited in most jurisdictions. Several states have established driver regulations for snowmobile operation. This is particularly important with regard to children. A child or young teenager should not be permitted to operate a snowmobile any more than he or she is able to legally drive an automobile.

In an effort to get snowmobiles off roadways and to provide safe terrain over which to operate, many localities have developed snowmobile trail systems. These trails are maintained by public authorities and are kept free of obstacles, such as fences, wire, trees, and dangerous bumps. More such trails should be designed in those parts of the country where snowmobiling is popular.

Motorcycles

The motorcycle is a two-wheeled cycle which is operated by an engine with enough horsepower to run at speeds equivalent to motorized cars and trucks. It is used as a recreational vehicle by some people; for others it is a necessary means of transportation. Regardless of its use, there are a number of factors related to safety that must be understood when considering this motorized vehicle.

Simply mentioning the motorcycle will cause varying reactions among different people. To some a cycle's image is exciting, thrilling, and daring. The speed and the power in one's hands gives a sense of exhilaration. To others, a motorcycle provides an economical source of transportation. For others, the motorcycle is a machine that causes noise and disruption of an otherwise quiet neighborhood.

There are a little more than four million registered motorcycles in operation in the United States.[1] Ninety percent of motorcycle operators are male, and most are under the age of 25.

Motorcycles are commonly used on both major highways and other lesser-traveled public roads. They also are operated as off-road vehicles. When driving on a public roadway, the motorcycle operator must obey all of the laws and regulations for the operation of any motor vehicle. Most states require a license to operate a motorcycle on public roadways. However, there is evidence that many drivers of motorcycles operate their cycles without a license. It has been reported that nearly one-half the motorcycle drivers who are either killed or who become involved in crashes did not have possession of a valid motorcycle operators' license at the time of the collision.[2]

As a recreational vehicle, off-road use of the motorcycle can take place in woods, over open country fields, in the desert or mountains, as well as in suburban housing developments. When a motorcycle is ridden in such off-road environments, care must be taken not to drive into objects lying across the trails. Stones, sticks, or logs stretched across the pathway will upset the cycle and can easily throw the rider. Fencing presents a particular hazard for the rider of an off-road cycle.

Motorcycle Collisions

It has been reported that in 1992 about 2,700 fatalities occurred among motorcycle riders.[3] In addition the National Highway Traffic Safety Administration reported that more than 66,000 injuries resulted from the operation of motorcycles in a given year.[4]

The motorcyclist involved in a collision has a much greater chance of being killed than does an individual riding in a four-wheel motor vehicle such as a car or truck. This stems from the lack of protection available to the driver or rider of a motorcycle who becomes involved in a collision.

Motorcycle injuries can occur to all parts of the body. Head injuries are the leading cause of fatality in motorcycle crashes. Injury also occurs to the arms and legs, as well as the chest and abdomen. Almost all motorcycle incidents lead to multiple injury that includes abrasions, lacerations, and fractures. Another motorcycle-related injury is "motorcycle burn"—a first- or second-degree burn, generally on the legs, resulting from contact with the exhaust pipe.

Motorcyclists should take measures to protect themselves in case of a crash. Gloves, jackets, long trousers, and boots provide a degree of protection against scrapes, bruises, abrasions, and other injuries. Face shields, goggles, and windshields can provide an important measure of protection against insects, small dirt particles, and other objects that can strike the face and the eyes.

Helmets

Because of the potential danger to the head in a motorcycle collision, the question of requiring anyone riding a cycle to wear a helmet has been strongly debated. There is little question that the helmet has played an important role in reducing the incidence and severity of injuries to the head.

However, mandating helmet use has been a very controversial issue. By the mid-1970s all but three states had implemented mandatory helmet-use laws. However, opposition arose by many motorcyclists, as well as others concerned about governmental regulation of one's individual rights. As a result of litigation and public pressure many states have rescinded, or greatly modified, these motorcycle helmet laws.

Those who are opposed to wearing helmets suggest that surrounding noises cannot be heard and that peripheral vision is impaired. Certainly noises may be muffled to some degree. However, it would seem that the alert motorcycle rider can learn to compensate for this. The noise generated by some motorcycles is such that it must be questioned how much surrounding traffic can be heard at all by the rider.

As with other issues where preventive measures are mandated, many have questioned whether it is appropriate by law to require individuals to wear helmets. These individuals suggest that any such mandates infringe on one's freedom and individual rights. As a result, helmet laws have been challenged legally as being unconstitutional.

Today helmet-use legislation varies by state. Three states have no requirements for helmet usage. Twenty-three states require helmet use only for individuals in specific age groups or for passengers; in several

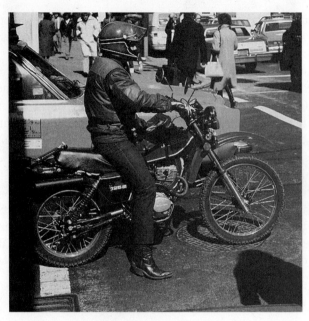

In spite of opposition by many motorcyclists to legal mandates requiring that helmets be worn, the evidence is overwhelming that helmets protect against serious injuries and many fatalities when involved in a collision.

cases, helmet possession but not usage is required. Universal usage of helmets for all riders is required in twenty-four states and in the District of Columbia.[5]

The importance of implementing legislation to mandate helmet use among motorcycle riders was noted in the recent federal health promotion/disease prevention objectives for the nation.[6] The specific objective calls for all 50 states to establish mandatory motorcycle helmet-use laws by the year 2000. For this objective to be achieved more than half of the states will need to develop and pass such legislation.

Licensure

Even though most states have some type of licensure regulations for operation of motorcycles, there is general feeling that better enforcement of these policies is needed. Supporting this call for enforcement is the fact that most motorcyclists involved in crashes do not have valid licenses.[7] All too often the operator was driving a cycle owned by another person.

Several measures for better licensing enforcement have been suggested.[8] One recommendation is that proof of possession of a valid license be required before an individual can purchase a motorcycle. Also, stiffer penalties for those who fail to comply with the law might help to reduce this problem.

Instruction in Motorcycle Operation

As with any motorized vehicle, every person who operates a motorcycle should possess skill in handling and operating the vehicle. Driving instruction should be available for anyone who seeks a motorcycle operator's license. No person should be permitted to operate a motorcycle who has not demonstrated basic minimal skills. Instruction in motorcycle operation seems to be as important for teenagers as is driver education instruction for operation of motor vehicles.

In an effort to improve the education of motorcyclists, the National Safety Council has added a two-hour supplement on motorcycle safety to its defensive driving course. This presentation covers basic information about the cycle, vehicle maintenance, riding rules and guidelines, and how to ride in differing weather conditions and in varying road and traffic environments. Similar motorcycle operator training programs are conducted by the individual states as well as by the Motorcycle Safety Foundation.[9] Such instructional programs should be helpful in reducing the number of motorcycle-caused fatalities and injuries.

Minibikes

The *minibike* is a small, two-wheeled motorized cycle with a gasoline-driven engine about the same size and power as that found on lawnmowers. Because minibikes usually have short wheelbases with rather small wheels, the result is an unstable vehicle, capable of reaching speeds of 20 to 30 miles per hour. Its potential hazards notwithstanding, the minibike is driven by increasing numbers of young children.

Several thousand persons a year receive hospital emergency room treatment for injuries resulting from the use of minibikes. Most of these are children 10 to 14 years of age. Parents often purchase these vehicles for their youngsters as young as 8 and 9. It is possible to purchase such vehicles with training wheels for children of preschool age.

The fact that many minibike operators are youngsters is one of the reasons that significant numbers of collisions result from their use as well as accompanying injuries. Many minibike operators perform dangerous maneuvers in an attempt to show off and gain attention. The practice of lifting the front wheel as one accelerates is common; jumping the vehicle over a barrier is another type of stunt that may lead to serious injury. Efforts must be taken to discourage these types of stunt activities.

Riding minibikes over uneven terrain can cause the operator to lose control of the vehicle and be thrown. Any person riding the minibike over open fields and through yards must be familiar with the terrain. Rocks, loose sand and gravel, and holes on the trail must be avoided, and the rider must stay away from fences stretched across these open spaces.

Injury often results to minibike riders from structural defects of the vehicle. Only sturdy, durable vehicles should be purchased. Minibikes with large wheels are much more stable than are those with smaller wheels. Unfortunately, most minibikes have smaller tires.

Brakes must be easy to apply. Many minibikes have only handbrakes which are not adequate, particularly for young riders. Minibikes should have a footbrake in combination with the handbrake, and riders should be given instruction in the use of both. It is not uncommon for the minibike rider to grab the throttle when attempting to apply the handbrake. The result can be tragic.

All minibike riders should wear protective clothing, including helmets. Too often the rider is seen driving around the neighborhood without a helmet. Safety education is essential.

Consideration for neighbors and small children must be taken by parents who purchase a minibike for their youngsters. The noise level of these vehicles must be controlled. Children should not be permitted to ride the minibike around in the yard if other houses are located nearby. Also, young minibike riders must be taught to keep their machines away from other small children. The 10-year-old who has a minibike and is executing stunts in the presence of a group of children to show off is creating a situation that has the potential for serious injury or worse.

Many minibike riders get their start when parents purchase a minibike to use in racing. In some localities minibike racing for children is a recreational activity. The reasonableness of such ''sporting events'' seems questionable. Those who feel this is an acceptable practice must be prepared to be responsible for and supervise their children's use of the minibike at all times. When children ride their minibikes improperly and in ways that are dangerous to themselves and others, the parents must be held responsible.

All-Terrain Vehicles (ATVs)

Another motorized vehicle that has been increasingly popular for recreational purposes, particularly in rural localities, is the *all-terrain vehicle* (ATV). The ATV is a small vehicle designed to travel on three or four low-pressure tires. It can achieve speeds of up to 40 miles per hour or more. Its basic construction makes it possible to travel at various rates of speed over many different types of terrain. It is able to go through sand, wet dirt, and water, up embankments, and through a variety of other settings.

In different locations around the country, areas have been set aside for the recreational operation of all-terrain vehicles. It is in these official parks, whether sand dunes or woods and forests, that conditions tend to be safe for the operation of these motorized recreational vehicles. Unfortunately, many people operate the machines in locations which are neither appropriate nor safe.

According to data of the Consumer Product Safety Commission, more than 85,000 injuries and over 200 fatalities occur annually that can be attributed to use of all-terrain vehicles. Nearly half of these fatalities involve operators under the age of 16.[10]

Particular concern has focused on the three-wheeled all-terrain vehicle which first began to be manufactured in the early 1970s. These vehicles tend to be much less stable than the four-wheeled model. In the case of any three-footed object, it is easy to shift the center of gravity—hence, to tip the object over. This also is true of the three-wheeled ATV.

As a result, in 1988 the Consumer Product Safety Commission banned the manufacture and sale of three-wheeled ATVs in the United States. It was the position of the Consumer Product Safety Commission that the safety and stability of these vehicles were not acceptable. However, any vehicles in operation at the time of the ban could still be used. At the time of the ban nearly a thousand deaths and hundreds of thousands of injuries had resulted from riding and operating three-wheeled ATVs—figures dating back to the vehicle's initial development and manufacture. The largest number of injuries that occurred while riding three-wheeler ATVs were face and scalp lacerations, fractures, concussions, and burns.[11]

Studies also have indicated that a major risk factor in ATV-related injuries and fatalities is the failure of the operators to wear helmets.[12] Only about one-third of ATV riders wear helmets. Unfortunately, helmet use is particularly low among children. It should be obvious that anyone riding these vehicles needs to wear personal protective equipment, such as boots, gloves, and trousers.

As with any recreational motorized vehicle, adequate training is vital. This is particularly the case for young people. No one should operate these vehicles without appropriate driver education. Included in these educational initiatives should be information about the laws and local ordinances that relate to the operation of all-terrain vehicles. The ATV Specialty Vehicle Institute of America has developed a training course for users. Training sites have been established and over a thousand instructors have been trained to conduct courses for ATV operators.

Outdoor Recreational Activities

There are innumerable recreational activities that people pursue out-of-doors, including a variety of individual sports. Each of these activities require specific motor skills, such as the ability to hit a golf ball, swing a tennis racket, or aim a croquet ball.

Another category of outdoor activities is that of formally organized or informal group recreational team sports. These include playing basketball, soccer, and softball on a spontaneous basis or in various types of recreational leagues. Volleyball is another team sport that is highly popular, particularly on the beach.

There are other kinds of recreational outlets for people out-of-doors. For some, horseback riding provides many opportunities for enjoyment. Among the elderly a game of shuffleboard is a time for social interaction and physical activity. As one can understand, it would be impossible to discuss completely all such recreational pursuits from the perspective of safety and injury prevention in the context of this chapter. Three outdoor recreational activities have been selected for further discussion in which people of various ages commonly participate. These will provide examples of the many issues and concerns which present themselves when considering outdoor recreational pursuits.

Camping

Thousands of Americans spend time camping in the out-of-doors every year. At one time camping was an activity reserved for scouting groups, a few young individuals hiking in the wilderness, and soldiers in the military. It was rare for a family to spend a vacation or even a long weekend on a camping trip in the forest or the mountains. Camping in the past usually involved carrying a small tent and a few necessities for cooking. The equipment used was not highly specialized.

Today camping has become a highly developed recreational activity for a large segment of the American population. Modern camping equipment is manufactured and sold in all types, colors, and price ranges. For example, many different kinds of motor vehicles can be purchased for camping purposes. One may choose to camp in a large self-propelled motor home with nearly all the necessities of a conventional household: television, inside plumbing facilities, built-in stereos, and comfortable beds. For others, camping means taking a lightweight tent on a backpacking trip into the mountains and sleeping on a canvas mattress unrolled onto the ground. Regardless of the type of camping experience, interest in camping has grown so that it is often difficult to find a quiet camping location on a weekend at many of America's favorite resort areas and state and national park campgrounds.

Camping, while enjoyable, holds many possibilities for injury and even fatality. The most common camping-related accident involves fire—especially some combination of campfires, stoves or lanterns, sleeping bags and tents. Even though most tents and sleeping bags are manufactured to be fireproof, campers must take every precaution to prevent a fire from occurring. Fires from campfires should be extinguished before people go to sleep.

Another danger associated with camping is the presence of carbon monoxide where camping heaters, lamps, and similar equipment is used. Care must be taken to provide sufficient fresh air circulation to guard against asphyxiation. It also would be wise to have a monitoring instrument available to warn when dangerous levels of carbon monoxide develop.

Being out-of-doors exposes people to numerous objects and situations that can result in injury. Cuts, bruises, and fractures often result from activities associated with the camping experience. Exposure to poisonous plants and other toxic agents can cause problems. Insect bites may not only disrupt an enjoyable camping experience, but may cause serious harm to the skin of people allergic to such toxins, respiratory problems, and even fatalities. Before going on a trip, campers should obtain a well-stocked emergency aid kit that, in turn, should be readily available for use in any circumstance.

Hunting

Most humans no longer have to hunt for their food supply, in order to obtain their clothing, or to provide for their shelter. Agriculture and manufacturing fulfill these needs in industrial societies. Instead of being essential for human survival, hunting today is a recreational pursuit for thousands of individuals. For example, an estimated half million deer hunters move into the woods and forests of northern Michigan and Wisconsin each fall. Thousands of duck hunters spend hours in cold, wet surroundings waiting for the chance to "bag their limit." Many individuals travel into wilderness areas in order to hunt and kill big game.

Although most hunters probably perceive themselves to be healthy and vigorous individuals, many die every year in situations resulting from their hunting experience. Many of these fatalities are not related to the use of firearms. Rather, they occur due to heart attacks.

People planning to go into the fields or the woods on a hunting expedition should learn to protect their personal physical well-being. Hunting usually necessitates much more vigorous physical activity than an individual normally performs in the course of daily activities. A reasonable degree of physical fitness is needed for the hunting experience. Every person planning to go hunting should participate in some physical conditioning prior to the opening of the hunting season. It is not out of the question to suggest that certain individuals should undergo a cardiovascular medical checkup before undertaking a hunting trip.

Far too many fatalities and injuries result from the use of firearms during hunting. The National Safety Council indicates that approximately 1,400 fatalities occurred in a recent year from the accidental use or misuse of firearms in recreational activities.[13] An undisclosed number of these incidents involved hunters.

Firearm safety must be practiced by every hunter. This, of course, is not only for the protection of one's own life and well-being, but also for the sake of other individuals in the fields or woods. It is essential to know how to handle the firearm in a safe manner.

Firearms should always be handled as if they were loaded. This means that even when one is sure that a particular weapon is not loaded, it should be handled as if it were. This basic guideline calls for pointing the muzzle of the weapon in a safe direction at all times. It should never be aimed toward people, houses, barns, or domestic livestock. When the *action* or working mechanism of a firearm is open, others can see that the weapon is unloaded. This precautionary measure should be maintained except when actually shooting at game.

Even though it might be easier to keep a firearm loaded, there are times when it is necessary to unload the gun. For example, when climbing a fence, crossing a log in a body of water, or climbing a tree, particular care must be given to carrying the weapon—or perhaps even better, actually unloading the firearm.

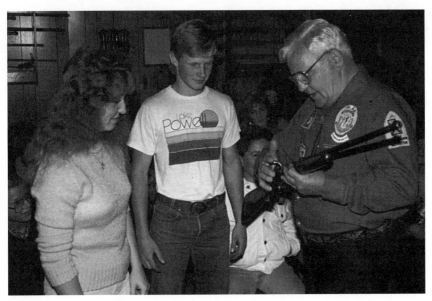

No one should go hunting who does not understand and practice safe handling of a firearm. Instructional programs for new hunters can be very useful in providing information that will help in the safe handling of a firearm.

In order to help make hunters more safety conscious and to provide basic instruction in hunting safety, some states require attendance at hunting safety courses before an individual is given a hunting license. The National Rifle Association offers hunter safety training courses. The emphasis of these programs is on the personal responsibility of the hunter for safety while hunting.

Regardless of how many safety precautions the hunter takes, accidental shootings do occur. Hunters should always carry appropriate first aid material in their hunting gear. They should go out in groups and leave word with someone where they plan to be.

Skiing

Throughout the northern and western Mountain States, New England, and in the mountains of the Appalachian region of the United States skiing, both downhill and Nordic, has become a popular recreational activity. New ski resorts, cross-country trail systems, and other facilities for skiing have been developed. Skiing is a big business in many communities in the United States.

With increasing numbers of people skiing, it is logical to expect that there will be an increase in the number of fatalities and injuries. The National Safety Council reports that there were 41 fatalities related to snow skiing during 1992.[14] Most fatalities result from collision with various objects, particularly trees. Speed and loss of control are major factors in such skiing accidents.

As with any individual recreational activity, the greater one's experience with snow skiing, the less the possibility there is of an injury occurring. The beginning skier has a much greater chance of being injured than does the experienced, expert skier. For this reason, a person should not venture out onto the ski slopes or into the woods on a cross-country ski run until receiving proper instruction in safety measures.

Skiing injuries also can be reduced by appropriate physical conditioning. As with all strenuous activities, the better one's physical condition, the less the likelihood of injury.

When on a ski slope, certain courtesies must be observed. The skier should never stop on the slope. This action blocks the path and can lead to a collision when the next skier descends. It also is courteous to inform a skier when he or she is being overtaken by another person on the slope.

Along with proper instruction, training, and courtesy, the type of equipment used is vital to injury prevention. It is estimated that 80 percent of ski injuries occur to the leg. For this reason, particular attention should be given to the choice of boots and the ski bindings.

Boots must fit properly and be comfortable. Ski boots today are designed with both safety and comfort in mind. Ski bindings are designed to release when the individual falls. However, many leg injuries in skiing result from improper functioning of these bindings. When the skier loses control and falls, the bindings should release; yet bindings must not release too easily or they can cause a fall.

Ski bindings are exposed to a number of potentially harmful environmental conditions. Dirt, ice, salt, and vibration all have an effect on bindings. Every skier must take precautions to protect bindings from wear and damage.

The first line of aid for injured skiers usually is the National Ski Patrol, a voluntary rescue organization that had its beginnings in 1936. The objective of the National Ski Patrol is to get the injured person out of the cold and to a hospital, preventing further injury or exposure to the elements. Members of the National Ski Patrol must undergo a training program that includes the American Red Cross course and a skiing and toboggan-handling course, as well as service for a probationary period.

The activities of the National Ski Patrol not only include rendering emergency services to the injured skier, but its personnel also become involved in the search and rescue of lost skiers. Danger to skiers often exists when avalanche conditions are present in an area. At most ski resorts warnings are posted when conditions are dangerous for normal skiing. However, all too often these warnings are ignored, and individuals become trapped or lost.

With increased interest in Nordic—also known as cross-country skiing—more individuals have become lost, injured, or fatigued and dehydrated in remote areas. Isolated skiers as well as winter hikers often have been rescued by Ski Patrol personnel.

Cycling

The first bicycle was built sometime in the latter part of the eighteenth century.[15] It was a crude production in which a wooden bar was supported on two wheels while the operator sat in a padded saddle; the machine was propelled by the operator's feet pushing against the ground. Since then, significant improvements in bicycle construction have taken place, so that today one can find many kinds of bicycles with different gear ratios, tire sizes, and other features. A consumer may purchase a two-wheel bicycle for as little as $50 to $75 or as much as several thousand dollars.

For most of the present century the bicycle has served as a recreational toy for children. Once people reached the age they could drive motor vehicles they seemed no longer as interested in riding a bicycle. Only rarely would an adult go out on the streets and roadways on a two-wheeler. The image of a mature man or woman wearing business clothes peddling down the street or going to work on a bicycle may have seemed incongruous, too unsophisticated, or trivial to the average American.

In the past several years, however, there has been a significant increase in bicycling activities throughout the United States. It no longer is unusual to see adults riding bicycles for recreational purposes or even as transportation for going to work.

Several sociological and economic factors account for this resurgence in bicycle riding. In the context of the growing concern about exercise for fitness and health reasons, the bicycle provides an excellent opportunity for aerobic exercise for many people.

For others, concern about the environment has led to increased interest in bicycle riding. Since the motor vehicle is a major contributor to air pollution, some individuals feel that there needs to be a reduction in the operation of motor vehicles. If one can ride a bike to work, to the store, or for other errands instead of driving an automobile, then a minor contribution is being made to improving the environment.

Economic reasons also are given as to why some people have taken to riding bicycles. Some people have used the bicycle as an alternative to motor-vehicle transportation in order to reduce their expenditures for fuel.

Even though there has been an increase in bicycling for these and other reasons, it is fair to suggest that in the United States most adults, and probably all children, continue to think of cycling as a recreational activity. Until improved bicycle pathways and local ordinances are developed that provide alternatives to riding bicycles in the flow of motor-vehicle traffic, it is unlikely that the bicycle will be used widely as a regular means of transportation in this country.

The general increase in bicycle riding activity has been a welcome development. However, along with the growth in numbers of cyclists there also has been an upswing in fatalities and injuries related to cycling.

Approximately 700 fatalities occur annually to bicycle riders; in addition, there are thousands of injuries requiring hospital or emergency medical service.[16] With more people riding bicycles today than ever before in history, the need increases for safety measures that reduce the likelihood of bicycle-related mishaps. The individual bicyclist must be alert at all times since there is no protection in a possible collision—particularly with a motor vehicle.

The Bicycle—a Toy or Not?

Is the bicycle a toy? Should it be regulated as such? Or do you view the bicycle as a vehicle of transportation? These questions have caused concern to the many adults who ride bicycles.

The Consumer Product Safety Commission has listed the bicycle as the most hazardous household product—classifying it as a household toy. Regulations governing safety factors and frame structure have been established by the Consumer Product Safety Commission under authority of the Consumer Product Safety Act which governs construction of children's toys. The commission defines a child as anyone 15 years of age or younger. Since 15-year-olds are able to ride adult-sized bicycles, all bicycles ought to be regulated under provisions governing the safety of children's toys according to the logic of these regulations. Many of the thousands of adults who use the bicycle as a means of transportation, as well as a recreational activity, take exception to the government's classification of the bicycle as a toy.

Cycle Construction and Operation

An important consideration in bicycle safety is to assure that the cycle is built solidly and that all parts are functioning properly. A bicycle that is in good operating condition must be adjusted to the size and fit of the rider.

There are several procedures or "checks" that a bicycle rider should make in determining whether the bicycle fits properly. The cyclist should be able to straddle the frame with both feet flat on the ground. If the individual cannot do this, then the bicycle frame is too large for the rider and a serious potential for injury exists. The saddle should be adjusted to a height that will permit the seated rider's heel to rest on the pedal with the leg completely extended. While pedaling the bicycle an individual should sit so that the ball of each foot is placed on the pedal with a slight bend at the knee.

The rider should be certain that the component parts of the cycle are functioning properly. Bolts must be secure and firm. No bicycle should be used in which the braking mechanism is faulty. The braking lever, cable, and brake blocks need to be checked frequently for proper operation. When riding the bicycle in wet weather, the rider should apply the brakes lightly from time to time to help dry out the braking blocks. Application of the brakes on a wet rim or block makes it very difficult to bring the bike to a rapid stop.

The wheels and tires of a bicycle need attention. Badly worn tires must be replaced. A common problem results when spokes are broken, causing the wheel to become misaligned. As a result, the cycle will not run "true" and becomes difficult to handle.

Bicycle handlebars should be level and secure. Many bicycles with high-rise handlebars have been purchased for children. This type of bicycle not only has high handlebars but it is usually accompanied by a long, banana-shaped seat with a backrest. The safety and handling of this type of bike has been debated by many safety officials.

Personal Gear

Because of the nature of bicycling there is little personal protective clothing that can be worn. However, 80 percent of all bicycle fatalities and two-thirds of hospital admissions resulting from cycling are the result of head injuries.[17] Wearing a helmet can reduce the risk of head injury by as much as 85 percent. It becomes obvious that the most important personal safety equipment that can be worn is the helmet. It also would seem logical to recommend that states and local governmental agencies develop legislation mandating the wearing of helmets while riding bicycles.

Most helmets sold currently consist of a hard plastic or fiberglass shell with a lining of expanded polystyrene foam. On impact the material crushes, absorbing the shock.

It does not take a lot of research studies to confirm the value of wearing helmets while cycling. Increasing numbers of serious recreational bicycle riders are wearing them. However, as with motorcyclists, a number of reasons are given for not wearing helmets. Some suggest that they are uncomfortable. Others out for just a short ride in the neighborhood do not consider that they will be involved in any situation in which an injury could occur.

Very few children wear helmets while riding their bicycles. Common reasons for not wearing them are that they are uncomfortable, they are expensive, and because of the influence of peer pressure. In some localities there are ordinances that require that infants riding in cycle seats must have helmets. However, since most children never wear helmets, adults have not developed the habit when riding their own bicycles.

It is extremely important that a cyclist is easily seen, especially at dusk or at night. Wearing reflective material and having reflectors on the wheels, seat, and cycle itself will help oncoming traffic to see the bicycle.

Rules of the Road

Every cyclist should know the rules of riding a bicycle on public streets and roads. Bicycles should be ridden on the right side of the street going with the flow of traffic. Many adults were taught as a child to ride a bicycle facing the traffic. This is inappropriate. Cyclists should also use hand signs and signals when turning.

While riding the bicycle it must be remembered that pedestrians have the right of way; also cyclists must be alert to road conditions. Even though the cyclist may have the right of way, this should never be contested with a motor vehicle involved. Obviously, the cyclist in such situations is risking serious injury or a fatality.

Falls occur with many cyclists at railroad crossings. The bicycle rider must always cross railroad tracks at ninety-degree angles. Otherwise it is possible to get the wheels of the bicycle caught in the tracks. The resulting fall may well injure the rider and damage the wheels and structure of the bicycle.

Public Playgrounds

Every day thousands of children play on public playgrounds throughout the nation. Some playgrounds are located in parks, others in public housing developments in the large urban cities, on school grounds, as well as on church grounds and in other public places. It is estimated that as many as 500,000 children are treated in hospital emergency rooms for injuries associated with playground equipment annually—a majority of them under 10 years of age. Most injuries are the result of falls from the equipment. Two-thirds of injuries occurred to the head and the neck.[18]

Since falls are the major type of injury it is important to consider the composition of the ground surface underneath the various play apparatus. The Consumer Product Safety Commission has concluded that asphalt, concrete, brick, blacktop, cinders, and packed earth are unsafe as surfaces for playgrounds. It is the recommendation of the commission that energy-absorbing surfaces should be used.[19] These include the use of rubber mats, wood chips, and sand. All playground equipment should be placed over such energy-absorbing surfaces.

There are numerous other factors that must be taken into consideration when developing a safe playground. Each type of play equipment demands special consideration. For example, hard, heavy swing seats can be particularly dangerous when they strike a child. Wood and metal swing seats should be replaced by rubberized seats for safety purposes. The moving parts of gliders and seesaws can pinch or crush the fingers of a child. Regardless of whether it is a swing, a slide, climbing equipment, or rotating equipment, all parts must be securely fastened and not be broken or malfunctioning.

The Consumer Product Safety Commission has identified several dangers that are found particularly with playground equipment.[20] The legs of all playground equipment must be securely anchored below ground level to avoid tripping. Measures must be taken to assure that there are no sharp edges at points where pieces of the equipment come together; screws and bolts used to hold the equipment together should not be exposed. Every piece of playground equipment must be installed so as to provide a minimum of 6 feet of space from any obstructions, such as fences, buildings, walkways, poles, and trees.

In order to improve playground safety it is necessary to check the safety of the equipment on a regular basis. In 1991 the Consumer Product Safety Commission published guidelines for public playground equipment. This document contains recommendations that can serve as a guideline for inspecting the equipment found on a playground.

Measures must be instituted to remove and replace all broken parts and equipment as soon as such defects are noted. This can only be accomplished by routine, systematic site inspections. Also, children should receive instruction as to the proper way to use all playground equipment.[21]

The importance of providing and maintaining a safe playground environment was emphasized in court litigation in 1992. A court in the District of Columbia rendered a multimillion-dollar settlement to the family of a boy who was injured after falling on his head on the asphalt surface underlying an arched climber. The long-term impact of this litigation remains to be seen. Should there be increased multimillion-dollar court settlements in the future, one wonders if communities and those who own property on which playgrounds are located will be likely to remove such equipment. Such actions would be most unfortunate for children.

Summary

Participation in recreational activities for Americans involves a variety of different options. Many individuals choose the use of motorized vehicles such as snowmobiles, motorcycles, minibikes, and all-terrain vehicles (ATVs).

Each of these recreational vehicles has the potential for serious injuries or could result in fatality. It is important that those who operate and ride on motorized recreational vehicles learn the rules of the road and ride accordingly. No person should venture out on a motorized recreational vehicle until adequate skills have been developed for the operation of that vehicle.

There are numerous other recreational activities which do not involve the operation of a motor vehicle. Camping, hunting, and skiing are examples of such activities that attract people of all ages and social groups. Most Americans participate in either individual or team recreational games of some type.

Bicycle riding is a popular recreational pursuit as well as a means of transportation for many adults. Generally, the streets and highway patterns in most communities do not lend themselves to the riding of bicycles. For this, and other reasons, it is important that safety measures be taken to assure that injury will not result from bicycle riding.

With all cycles—motorcycles, minibikes, bicycles, and all-terrain vehicles—it is important that all riders wear helmets to protect the head and face in case of a collision or fall. Mandating use of helmets has not been popular among many cycle riders. Yet this is the one most single important preventive measure that can be taken to reduce serious injury and fatality among cycle riders of all types.

Discussion Questions

1. Discuss some of the recreational appeal of the snowmobile.
2. What are some of the dangers linked to operation of a snowmobile?
3. Identify some of the major safety concerns associated with operation of a motorcycle.
4. What are some reasons given by those individuals who oppose mandatory helmet regulations for motorcyclists?
5. What are the rules in your state regarding licensure of motorcycle operators?
6. Explain safety factors associated with operation and use of the minibike.
7. What is the all-terrain vehicle (ATV)?
8. Discuss the action of the Consumer Product Safety Commission in banning the manufacture and sale of three-wheeled ATVs.
9. Explain safety measures that should be taken to prevent a firearm accident while hunting.
10. Give some reasons for the increased interest in both Nordic and downhill skiing in the United States.
11. What are ski bindings?
12. Explain the importance of the National Ski Patrol.
13. Describe measures that should be taken to assure that a bicycle is safe for operation before setting out on a ride.
14. Should bicycle riders be required to wear safety helmets? Defend your answer.
15. Discuss some of the precautions that should be taken to assure as safe a playground as possible.
16. What position has the Consumer Product Safety Commission taken regarding the ground surface underneath apparatus on a public playground?

Suggested Readings

"Bike Helmets: Unused Lifesavers." *Consumer Reports* 55, no. 5 (May 1990): 348–51.

Centers for Disease Control. "Alcohol Use and Horseback-Riding—Associated Fatalities—North Carolina, 1949–1989," *Morbidity and Mortality Weekly Report* 41, no. 19 (15 May 1992): 335–41.

———. "Carbon Monoxide Levels During Indoor Sporting Events—Cincinnati, 1992–1993," *Morbidity and Mortality Weekly Report* 43, no. 2 (21 January 1994): 21–23.

———. "Fatal Carbon Monoxide Poisoning in a Camper-Truck—Georgia," *Morbidity and Mortality Weekly Report* 40, no. 9 (8 March 1991): 154–55.

———. "Playground-Related Injuries in Preschool-Aged Children—United States, 1983–1987," *Morbidity and Mortality Weekly Report* 37, no. 41 (21 October 1988): 629–33.

Colburn, Nona, and others. "Should Motorcycles Be Operated Within the Legal Alcohol Limits for Automobiles," *The Journal of Trauma* 35, no. 2 (August 1993): 183–86.

Dannenberg, Andrew L., and others. "Bicycle Helmet Laws and Educational Campaigns: An Evaluation of Strategies to Increase Children's Helmet Use," *American Journal of Public Health* 83, no. 5 (May 1993): 667–74.

Ganos, Doreen, and others. "Trauma Associated With Three- and Four-Wheeled All-Terrain Vehicles: Is the Four-Wheeler an Unrecognized Health Hazard?" *American Surgeon* 54, no. 7 (July 1988): 429–33.

Gold, Seymour M. "Inspecting Playgrounds for Hazards," *California Parks and Recreation* 46, no. 4 (Winter 1990): 39–42.

Hamilton, Mark G., and Bruce I. Tranmer. "Nervous System Injuries in Horseback-Riding Accidents," *The Journal of Trauma* 34, no. 2 (February 1993): 227–32.

Kizer, Kenneth W. "Wilderness Emergencies: Be Prepared," *Emergency Medicine* 23, no. 8 (30 April 1991): 88–102.

Kraus, Jess F., and others. "Motorcycle Licensure, Ownership, and Injury Crash Involvement," *American Journal of Public Health* 81, no. 2 (February 1991): 172–76.

Lund, Adrian, and others. "Motorcycle Helmet Use in Texas," *Public Health Reports* 106, no. 5 (September–October 1991): 576–78.

McConkey, John Patrick. "When the Knee Goes Downhill," *Emergency Medicine* 24, no. 4 (15 March 1992): 324–31.

McDermott, Frank T., and others. "The Effectiveness of Bicyclist Helmets: A Study of 1710 Casualties," *The Journal of Trauma* 34, no. 6 (June 1993): 834–45.

McSwain, Norman E., and Anita Belles. "Motorcycle Helmets—Medical Costs and the Law," *The Journal of Trauma* 30, no. 10 (October 1990): 1189–99.

Otis, Joanne, and others. "Predicting and Reinforcing Children's Intentions to Wear Protective Helmets While Bicycling," *Public Health Reports* 107, no. 3 (May–June 1992): 283–89.

Pless, I. Barry, Rene Verreault, and Sonia Tenina. "A Case-Control Study of Pedestrian and Bicyclist Injuries in Childhood," *American Journal of Public Health* 79, no. 8 (August 1989): 995–98.

Pollack, Charles Victor, and Susan Baker Pollack. "Injury Severity Scores in Desert Recreational All-Terrain Vehicle Trauma," *The Journal of Trauma* 30, no. 7 (July 1990): 888–92.

Reid, David C., and others. "Spine Trauma Associated with Off-Road Vehicles," *The Physician and Sportsmedicine* 16, no. 6 (June 1988): 142–52.

Sacks, Jeffrey J., and others. "Evaluation of an Intervention to Reduce Playground Hazards in Atlanta Child-Care Centers," *American Journal of Public Health* 82, no. 3 (March 1992): 429–31.

Sosin, Daniel M., and others. "Head Injury Associated Deaths from Motorcycle Crashes," *Journal of the American Medical Association* 264, no. 18 (14 November 1990): 2395–99.

Thompson, R. S., F. P. Rivara, and D. C. Thompson. "A Case-Control Study of the Effectiveness of Bicycle Safety Helmets," *New England Journal of Medicine* 320, no. 21 (25 May 1989): 1361–67.

Wagle, Vithal G., and others. "Is Helmet Use Beneficial to Motorcyclists?" *The Journal of Trauma* 34, no. 1 (January 1993): 120–22.

Wallach, Frances. "Old Playgrounds, New Problems," *Parks and Recreation* 28, no. 4 (April 1993): 46–50, 91.

Wallach, Frances. "Playground Safety Update," *Parks and Recreation* (August 1990): 46–50.

Endnotes

1. National Safety Council, *Accident Facts, 1993 Edition* (Itasca, IL: National Safety Council, 1993), 68.
2. Jess F. Kraus and others, "Motorcycle Licensure, Ownership, and Injury Crash Involvement," *American Journal of Public Health* 81, no. 2 (February 1991): 172.
3. National Safety Council, *Accident Facts 1993,* 68.
4. Ibid.
5. Ibid.

6. Department of Health and Human Services, *Healthy People 2000: National Health Promotion and Disease Prevention Objectives,* (Washington, DC: U.S. Government Printing Office, 1991), 284.
7. Jess F. Kraus and others, "Motorcycle Licensure," 172.
8. Ibid.
9. Motorcycle Safety Foundation, 2 Jenner Street, Suite 150, Irvine, CA 92718.
10. Data are obtained from undated brochures of the Consumer Product Safety Commission.
11. Charles Victor Pollack and Susan Baker Pollack, "Injury Severity Scores in Desert Recreational All-Terrain Vehicle Trauma," *The Journal of Trauma* 30, no. 7 (July 1990): 889.
12. Ibid.
13. National Safety Council, *Accident Facts 1993,* 5.
14. Ibid., 92.
15. *Complete Bicycle Book* (Los Angeles: Petersen Publishing, 1972), 234.
16. National Safety Council, *Accident Facts 1993,* 79.
17. Joanne Otis and others, "Predicting and Reinforcing Children's Intentions to Wear Protective Helmets While Bicycling," *Public Health Reports* 107, no. 3 (May–June 1992): 283–89.
18. Centers for Disease Control, "Playground-Related Injuries in Preschool-Aged Children—United States, 1983–1987," *Morbidity and Mortality Weekly Report* 37, no. 41 (21 October 1988): 630.
19. U.S. Consumer Product Safety Commission, *A Handbook for Public Playground Safety: General Guidelines for New and Existing Playgrounds,* vol. 1 (Washington, DC: U.S. Consumer Product Safety Commission, 1986).
20. Ibid., 10–11.
21. Centers for Disease Control, "Playground-Related Injuries," 631.

CHAPTER 10

Water Safety

Chapter Outline

Introduction
Drowning
Swimming
  Open Bodies of Water
  Home Swimming Pools
  Community Swimming Pools
Boating
  Rules of the Water
  Specific Boating Safety Issues
  Handling Boat Capsizes
  Alcohol Consumption and Boating
  Nonmotorized Boating

Safety on the Ice
Other Water Activities
  Surfing
  Skin Diving
  Scuba Diving
  Water Skiing
Water Instruction Programs
Summary
Discussion Questions
Suggested Readings
Endnotes

Introduction

A body of water attracts people of all ages. A small pond or creek is a favorite play spot for young children. Lakes and oceans provide numerous recreational opportunities. Boats of all sizes and shapes navigate our rivers and lakes. So popular is swimming that thousands of homeowners have built swimming pools in their yards. Some type of water activity is to be found in nearly every national, state, or local park in the United States.

Not only are bodies of water used for recreational purposes, but thousands of people earn their livelihoods on and around them. Every day on the lakes and the oceans of the world people are involved in commercial fishing for their livelihood. Large boats carry wheat, coal, grain, steel, and hundreds of manufactured products throughout the Great Lakes and beyond through the St. Lawrence Seaway to hundreds of ports throughout the world. Extensive barge traffic on the nation's major river arteries transports many different products to ports along the rivers.

Millions of people go to the beach each year. Most of these people do not swim. They paddle around, sunbathe, or jump about in the waves. Visit the local swim club on a hot summer day, and you will see several hundred people in and around the pool. Most, however, will not be swimming. Take a trip to the shore, and you will find most individuals sunning, building sand castles, or beachcombing.

Bodies of water attract people not only in warm or hot weather, but also during the colder months. Ice skating, ice sailing, ice fishing, and other related winter pursuits bring people into contact with the water environment throughout the entire year.

Yet, despite the profitable or therapeutic value of exposure to bodies of water for play and work, thousands of people die annually from drowning and other water-related incidents. In addition, many more are injured in the water environment. Regardless of the water activity in which one engages, it is important to take safety measures. To be uninformed or unresponsive to safety issues may lead to catastrophe. One basic skill should be acquired by any person venturing forth onto a body of water—*the ability to swim.* Individuals also should be familiar with rules and regulations designed to prevent water-related catastrophes from occurring.

Many people play rather than swim because they do not possess either adequate swimming skill or endurance. Many have never had any swimming instruction. Only a few schools include swimming in the physical education curriculum. Young people may receive swimming instruction at camps or as part of such programs as scouting. Adults may have opportunities to learn to swim in adult education courses. Often the basic instruction given in these settings is just enough to make a person think that he or she is more competent than is really the case.

Drowning

The human organism cannot exist submerged under water for very long. In order for the body to function a continuous, fresh supply of oxygen is necessary. Without oxygen, suffocation occurs in a matter of minutes.

Approximately 4,300 drowning fatalities occur on an annual basis in the United States. At greatest risk for drowning are children under 5 years of age and males between the ages of 15 and 34.[1] A major factor impacting this latter population group is the involvement in boating activities and alcohol consumption.

After motor-vehicle fatalities, drownings are the leading cause of unintentional death between the ages of 1 and 44. The federal government has established the health promotion/disease prevention objective of reducing deaths from drowning from 2.1 per 100,000 to 1.3 per 100,000 by the year 2000.[2] In order to accomplish this objective three specific population groups have been targeted for program emphasis. These target populations are children under the age of 4, males between 15 and 34, and all African-American males.[3]

The National Centers for Disease Control and Prevention, in identifying priorities for injury control in the 1990s, called for increased research relating to drownings and near drownings that result in hospitalization.[4] Special attention should be given to drowning among minority populations. Also the report called for research concerning drownings associated with water other than in pools.

Many drownings occur in rivers and creeks. In these bodies of water, unsuspecting individuals often are caught in water currents and are unable to escape to safety. It is less likely for a drowning to occur at a crowded beach. One reason for this is the availability of lifeguards at most large beaches. Also, at crowded beaches most people do not swim a great deal. Instead they come to sunbathe, picnic, or walk along the water's edge.

More than a fourth of all drownings occur while the victim is participating in activities not normally considered to be dangerous.[5] These activities include such things as fishing from docks, bridges, or along the shore. It may involve playing, wading, or walking near the water. The important point to remember is that it is not necessary for there to be deep water for a drowning to take place. People drown in bathtubs as well as lakes, oceans, and streams.

The suddenness of most drownings makes coping with the tragedy very difficult. One moment the individual is active, alert, and enjoying the beauty of the water experience. The next moment the person is lost under the surface of the water. Such experiences are traumatic for parents, relatives, and friends. The importance and need for effective supervision of all swimming activities to protect against drowning cannot be overemphasized.

Concern about childhood drownings has been an ongoing emphasis of the United States Consumer Product Safety Commission. In the early 1990s safety alerts were issued regarding hazards for drowning in toilets (usually the result of the child falling into the toilet headfirst) and in large buckets (the five-gallon bucket was noted as a particular danger), and for drowning as a result of children left unattended in bathtubs while sitting in baby ''supporting ring'' devices. There have been fatalities associated with all of these situations. The Consumer Product Safety Commission strongly endorsed the need to keep children away from any water container and to supervise young children in bathtubs at all times, regardless of how protected it is felt the child may be.

Alcohol consumption is associated with as many as 50 percent of adult drownings. As a result, alcohol should not be used by anyone operating a boat, fishing, or participating in other water activities. Individuals who have been drinking heavily should not be permitted to venture out onto a body of water. Neither should one who has been drinking alcohol swim in the backyard pool.

Everyone, regardless of the ability to swim, should take preventive measures when riding in boats or when involved in other water-related activities. Water skiers should wear life jackets. Immediate availability of life jackets is required in most states for people riding in boats. Small children should be required to wear life jackets at all times while in a boat.

Swimming

People swim in a variety of different settings—pools, ponds, rivers, lakes, and oceans. When swimming in any body of water, it is important that the person is aware of the depth of the water. Every swimming area should be free of debris such as glass, cans, logs, and rocks. The swimmer must know what kind of bottom is present, as the slope and the footing are important in preventing an unintentional injury or fatality. Specific water environments also may require unique safety knowledge and practices.

Open Bodies of Water

Extreme caution must be taken when swimming or diving into open bodies of water such as shallow lakes, ponds, streams, or rivers. The path of the dive should be planned. Failure to do so can cause the diver to strike underwater objects, leading to serious crippling head and neck injuries.

Whenever one swims in a river or at the seashore, there can be dangers from the various currents and tides. The current of a flowing stream or river can catch swimmers by surprise and pull them under the water or dash them against rocks before they have time to react.

Undertow is a type of current resulting from the breaking of waves upon a beach. The wave breaks over the beach and then recedes back toward the lake or ocean. If the waves are large enough and the beach has a slope, the undertow will have great force that can pull a person out into the water. If a swimmer is caught in such a current, he or she should not "fight" the water. It is best to be led by the current until an object such as a tree limb can be grabbed or until the current recedes.

Home Swimming Pools

There is no reliable estimate of the number of people that have home swimming pools. In parts of the country such as California, Florida, and most of the other states in the south, many homes have pools. Home swimming pools may be large and permanently built into the ground. On the other hand, many are the above-the-ground type. Any type of home swimming pool presents the possibility for drowning and injuries.

It is estimated that as many as 500 fatalities occur annually in home swimming pool drownings.[6] The Consumer Product Safety Commission also estimates that there are about 3,000 near drownings in home swimming pools each year that require hospital emergency room treatment and that involve children under 5 years of age.[7]

Many instances of drowning and injuries in home swimming pools could be prevented if several basic safety precautions are taken. As many as half the number of drownings can be eliminated if there is always adult supervision while a home pool is in use and if the pool is enclosed properly. The Centers for Disease Control and Prevention recommend that four-sided isolation fencing of at least five feet in height with self-closing latches should be required of all home pools.[8]

Contrary to the thinking of many people, drowning victims normally do not call for help or thrash about. Often they will quietly disappear below the surface of the water. For this reason, it is important to be alert around a pool, particularly in supervising children.

All local ordinances and regulations must be adhered to in constructing a home swimming pool. Because people, particularly small children, must be kept away from the pool when there is no supervision, it is wise to enclose a pool with a fence sufficiently high to prevent people from climbing over and falling into the water. A fence enclosure should have a gate that self-closes and a latch that locks. It would seem logical that mandatory fencing and gates around home swimming pools, both in-ground and above-ground, should be public policy. Another reason for adherence to local ordinances in the construction of a home swimming pool is the legal responsibility that one must assume in having such a facility on personal property.

Not only should preventive measures be taken, but the home swimming pool industry itself should be encouraged to consider safety in the construction and sale of their products.[9] Injury prevention technology might include development of energy-absorbing pool bottoms to reduce the possibility of diving related injuries.

Community Swimming Pools

There are many community swimming pools in America's cities, many of them municipal pools in parks and community buildings. Others are private swim clubs open to public memberships. These pools often are large enough to accommodate many people, with sections for small children to play in the water along with depths that are sufficient for diving.

Many swimming pool injuries result from falling on slippery decks, ladders, and diving boards. Nonslip material should be used on the deck areas surrounding a pool. A diving board and all ladders also must be coated with nonslippery material. Even when such material is used in the construction of a pool, all occupants and users of the pool should be warned about running on the deck. Any type of horseplay near a swimming pool may be the cause of serious injury.

Diving boards present a particular hazard around swimming pools. There should be at least eight feet of water under a one-meter diving board. There also should be sufficient water depth for the diver to swim about after completing the dive. Many motel and apartment complex pools fail to provide safe depths at the diving end of their pools. Never dive into a pool until there is complete assurance that the water is deep enough so that the diver will not hit the bottom. Obviously that depth may vary according to the skill, age, and size of the swimmer.

Water slides can provide a thrill, particularly for children. However, extreme caution should be taken in using water slides. The person should slide sitting down, legs first. Entering the water head first may be exciting, but one can very easily hit the bottom of the pool and be seriously injured.

No pool should be constructed with underwater protrusions such as pipes. Pipes should be flush with the walls and the bottoms of the pool. If a pool is to be used at night, underwater lighting should be installed and grounded.

Care should be taken with electrical construction around a swimming pool. Electrical work is safer when completed by a licensed electrical contractor. Measures must be taken to protect against electrical shock to the pool users. Electrical appliances should not be used near a swimming pool. For example, a radio can easily fall into the water and electrocute swimmers.

Rescue equipment, including ring buoys and long poles, should be available at all swimming pools. Not only must such equipment be properly located where people can get them within a minimum of time, but everyone should have an understanding of the most effective ways in which they are to be used.

Boating

Pleasure boating attracts millions of people each year. The United States Coast Guard estimates that more than 10 million pleasure boats are registered in the country: inboard and outboard motorboats, motorized rowboats, motorized canoes, jet skis, and houseboats as well as canoes, paddleboats, sailboats, and nonmotorized rowboats. Each kind of boat provides specific experiences. The motorboat provides a feeling of excitement and exhilaration. On the other hand, a canoe provides a tranquil experience as the canoeists paddle along a quiet stream; a sailboat places the individual at the disposal of the winds of nature. Regardless of the kind of boating activity, each demands specific safety practices.

It is estimated that more than 60,000 recreational boating accidents occur each year. A National Transportation Safety Board recreational boating study reported 478 fatalities in 1993.[10] Seventy-one percent of these fatalities occurred when individuals were involved with motorized power boats. About one-half of these involved the use of alcohol. The economic costs associated with boating accidents amounted to as much as $100 million.

There is no substitute for receiving proper instruction in the operation of a boat. The more one knows about the boat and how it

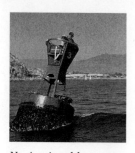

Navigational buoys are found along all waterways. Some are large so that they can be seen at long distances by big boat operators; others rely also on battery lighting systems or audible signals.
U.S. Coast Guard, 2100 Second Street, SW, Washington, DC 20593-0001.

operates, the greater the probability of having a safe experience. Motor boating enthusiasts do not tend to have adequate instruction in necessary safety procedures. Most people feel that if they can start an engine and steer the boat, as they do an automobile, that nothing further is necessary in order to operate the boat.

In 1994 Alabama became the first state to mandate licensing for operators of recreational boats. The law gave boat owners and operators five years to get a license. In order to obtain a license an individual must pass a written test covering boating safety and etiquette. People over the age of 40 do not have to pass the test in order to be licensed. There is no requirement that the person pass any kind of test of boat driving skills. It remains to be seen if other states develop and implement similar legislation.

Some states require that children under certain ages who are operating a boat be supervised by an individual over the age of 16. Also it is required in some states that individuals under certain ages must have completed a boat safety instruction course before they can operate a motorized boat. In 1988 the state of Maryland became the first state to implement a mandatory education program for youthful boat operators. Individuals up to the age of 21 must take an approved boating safety course. However, without any mandated tests for skill and knowledge of the rules for adults, it seems all the more important that people of all ages should be encouraged to take part in boating safety classes.

Rules of the Water

There are a number of rules of courtesy and safe operation—especially regarding yielding and right of way—that the operator of a boat should learn. For example, any boat being overtaken and passed by another boat has the right of way. It is important that the boat operator knows the meanings of the various buoys, the floating signposts for the boat operator. Buoys will be found in various shapes, colors, numbers, and configurations. Each buoy characteristic has a specific meaning, such as marking a danger area in the water. When traveling upstream, green buoys should be on the left or port side and red ones on the right or starboard side. One should never moor the boat on a navigational buoy. To do so is a federal offense subject to a monetary penalty.

Many boat operators do not realize that they are responsible for the wake that is made by their boats. One case in which a man lost his balance while getting out of the boat onto a dock is worth noting. As the individual was balancing with one foot still in the boat and the other on the dock, the boat began to rock in the water and the man was crushed between the boat and dock. The operator of a passing boat was held negligent because the boat he was driving exceeded the posted speed limit; the court ruled that the wake created by the passing boat caused the rocking of the boat from which the man fell.

The boat operator, or skipper, is completely responsible for the safe operation of the boat. The skipper of any boat must be well informed concerning the various handling characteristics of the craft and possess the skills to maintain control of the boat.

Boaters should be familiar with the various distress signals. This knowledge is useful when in need of assistance or when spotting another boat in need of help.

Specific Boating Safety Issues

Every boat should be equipped properly for safe operation and occupants should know how to deal with common emergency situations.

Equipment

There should be an anchor and line, strong and sufficient lines for tying the boat, oars, life preservers, and emergency repair tools on board every boat before casting off from shore. In addition, there should be flares, a foghorn, whistle, flashlight, first aid kit, and a bailing bucket on board. A compass and chart of the area must be considered standard equipment. All too often boat owners have only the required minimum amount of safety gear on board. For example, on a 16- to 25-foot powerboat only one fire extinguisher is required by law. Yet one needs more than the protection of a single fire extinguisher. Time is vital when a fire breaks out on these types of boats and multiple extinguishers may be essential.

Whenever operating a boat on a large lake, along the coasts, or on other major bodies of water, the occupants should have a marine radio on board. This radio can provide communication back to shore, can inform the persons on board of bad weather, can inform the Coast Guard of dangerous conditions, or can signal for help in an emergency.

Occupancy

Anyone getting into a boat should know how to step in without upsetting the boat or falling. Too many boating accidents result from overloading, so care should be taken to assure that only the proper number of individuals is permitted in the boat. Passengers should never stand up in a pleasure boat while it is in operation.

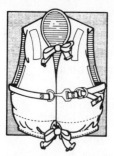
Off-shore life jacket
(Type I PFD)

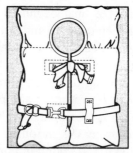
Near-shore buoyant vest
(Type II PFD)

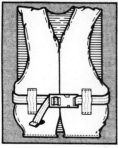
Flotation aid
(Type III PFD)

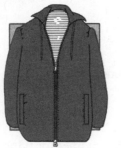

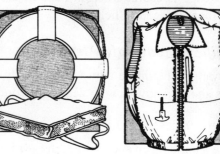
Throwable device
(Type IV PFD)

Inflated hybrid
(Type V hybrid device)

Several different types of flotation devices are available. Different factors determine which device is most useful considering the person and water conditions.
Source: U.S. Coast Guard.

Personal Flotation Devices

It is important that boat occupants wear *life jackets* or PFDs *(personal flotation devices)*. The United States Coast Guard rules require one PFD on board for each individual in the boat. Children should be required to wear PFDs and have them adjusted properly for their size.

There are different types of personal flotation devices. Selection of the particular device will depend upon the water conditions that will be encountered and the individual for whom it is designed to be used. Not only is it important to know how to properly use a personal flotation device, care must be taken to assure there are no rips, tears, or holes in it before going out on the water. Inflatable toys and rafts should never be used in place of personal flotation devices.

Types of Flotation Devices

Type I   (Off-Shore Life Jacket)—best for rough, open water in situations where rescue may be delayed. Turns the face of an unconscious individual up in the water.

Type II (Near-Shore Buoyant Vest)—useful in calm, inland lakes where rescue is imminent. Will not turn victim face up in the water. Less bulky than the Type I and more comfortable.

Type III (Flotation Aid)—useful in calm, inland water where rescue is imminent. Comfortable, comes in many styles (vests, coats, etc.). No support for the head.

Type IV (Throwable Device)—cushions, rings, and buoys that can be thrown to an individual in the water. Often used as seat cushions in boats.

Type V (Inflated Hybrid)—available in special varieties for such activities as boardsailing and water skiing.

Protection From Storms

A boater must be alert to weather patterns and not venture out onto a large body of water in stormy conditions. It is important to have some knowledge about potential weather and to be prepared to take measures to get to safety. When caught in a storm one should attempt to go to the nearest shore for protection.

Along many shorelines storm signals are flown by the Coast Guard when weather is inappropriate for pleasure craft. The recreational boater should be aware of the various storm signals and heed them. In addition, it would be useful to carry a transistor radio on a boat for receiving weather reports—a practice especially necessary on a large body of water.

Night Operation

Whenever a boat is used at night, it should be well lighted with navigational lights so that the boat can be seen from all directions while on the water. Only experienced sailors should venture out at night in a boat. Operators need to understand the light color system to determine the direction other boats are going.

Fire

Care must be taken to protect against fire aboard a boat. Never smoke while refueling, and make sure that the gasoline vapors do not settle in the lower parts of the boat (a natural tendency because such fumes are heavier than air). Hence, it is wise to ventilate all parts of the boat after fueling. Ventilation also is important when starting up the boat after it has been sitting for a lengthy period of time, such as overnight. Also, check the fuel line periodically to ensure that there are no fuel line leaks.

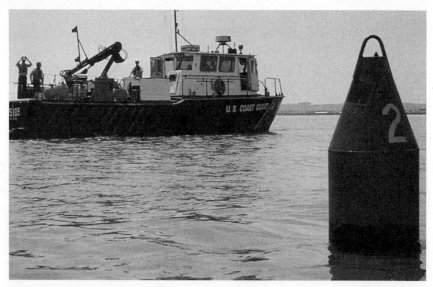

(a)

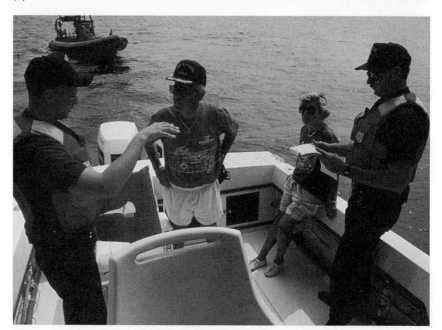

(b)

The U.S. Coast Guard carries out numerous tasks to assure safety on America's waterways. (a) They place and maintain buoys that mark the waterways and identify dangerous underwater objects. (b) Also, individual boat operators may be stopped to assure that there is appropriate equipment on board, such as PFDs and fire extinguishers.
Courtesy of: U.S. Coast Guard, 2100 Second Street, SW, Washington, DC 20593–0001.

Instruction

Boating can be an interesting and exciting recreational pursuit. Before launching out onto the water, however, boaters must take those measures that ensure safety, including instruction in navigational procedures and safety.

Handling Boat Capsizes

If a boat capsizes, should the occupant stay with the boat or attempt to swim to shore? There is no one answer that can be given for all circumstances, but if the boat continues to float, then it probably is wise to stay with the overturned boat. A capsized boat is easier to locate by another boat or a rescue plane than is an individual swimmer. Attempts to swim to shore often fail because the swimmer does not have sufficient skill or endurance.

Another important consideration at the time of a boating accident is the temperature of the water. If the water is cold, this will add to the difficulty of swimming to shore. Most people are comfortable swimming in water between 70 and 80 degrees Fahrenheit. When exposed to colder water, the body must work to maintain normal body temperatures. When combined with the need to produce energy for swimming, this added energy output can quickly lead to serious fatigue, exhaustion, and unconsciousness. Decreased body temperature, a consequence of cold water swimming, is a significant cause of death. It has been shown that immersion in cold water causes delirium; unconsciousness occurs and eventually death. Relative proficiency of a swimmer is not an issue in these circumstances.

Alcohol Consumption and Boating

The consumption of alcohol is a contributing factor to as many as half of all boating fatalities.[11] Alcohol impairs people's skills related to operation of a boat as well as their judgment. Alcohol can impact one's sense of balance or vision, both of which are vital when operating a boat on the water. Alcohol also creates a sensation of warmth which leads people to stay in cold water longer than if they were sober. Alcohol also impairs ability to swim, it shortens the cold water survival time, and it compounds the effects of wind, sun, and fatigue.

Because of the increase in boating collisions resulting from use of alcohol by the operator and occupants of the boat, most states have passed alcohol and boating laws designed to reduce the use of alcohol among boaters. Most regulations set standards for intoxication while operating a boat. These blood alcohol concentration (BAC) levels are

0.10 percent for recreational vessels in most states. The Coast Guard has established 0.04 percent BAC levels for commercial boat operation.

Some jurisdictions now routinely check boaters for the presence of alcohol. In jurisdictions where there are such laws, boating deaths have dropped. The implied consent regulations have application to boaters in several states—i.e., refusal to take sobriety tests can be used against the boater in court.

Measures need to be implemented to restrict the sale as well as consumption of alcoholic beverages in boating areas. Greater sanctions should be leveled against drunken boat operators. Any boating safety program must include educating the public about the dangers of alcohol consumption and boat operation.

Nonmotorized Boating

Thousands of people enjoy boating activities in nonmotorized boats. Canoeing and sailing are the most common activities involving boats without motors.

As in any type of recreational activity, an individual must learn the basic skills of operating a canoe before venturing out on a body of water. No more than three people should ever be in a canoe at the same time. Lifejackets are mandated in most states for all occupants of a canoe. When canoeing on white-water rivers it is important that a helmet be worn to protect against injuries to the head should the canoe capsize and the occupants strike rocks or other debris along the stream. The degree of difficulty of the river should be known before attempting to negotiate a rapids by canoe. People must not attempt to go through a rapids that is too difficult for their individual abilities.

Sailboats come in a variety of sizes and styles. Operation of such boats is dependent upon the amount of wind that is available. A principal safety consideration is to possess the skill required to operate the sailboat safely and in specific conditions. One must be aware of weather conditions before venturing out on a body of water in a sailboat. As with motorized boats there is certain safety equipment that must be on board whenever taking such a boat out onto the water.

Safety on the Ice

Thousands of people make use of ice in winter for recreational purposes: ice skating, ice sailing, snowmobiling, and ice fishing. The activity may be as hazardous as a child walking on thin ice covering a neighborhood pond or as relatively safe as a community ice festival with thousands of motor vehicles being driven out onto strong, solid ice. Regardless of the activity or the numbers of people involved, it is necessary to emphasize safety on the ice.

The safety of ice depends for the most part on its thickness as well as whether it is solid or chipped or cracked. If ice is broken, yet is reasonably thick, there is danger of being stranded on an ice floe that breaks away and moves to some other part of the river or lake. Ice that is one inch thick or less should not be used for any recreational pursuit. When ice is two inches thick, it is safe only for one person. It is best to stay off ice with this thickness. Ice that is three inches thick will support a small group of people in a single file. Ice that is four inches or more is usually safe for such activities as skating, sledding, or ice fishing.

When a person has fallen into water through the ice, emergency rescue procedures must be employed immediately. The individual who falls through the ice will often grab at the edge and attempt to climb out of the water. This is a natural reaction but a dangerous procedure because that person's weight will break the edge of the ice and the victim will fall back into the water. It is better for the individual to kick the legs as in swimming, lifting the lower part of the body; the arms should be stretched forward over the ice. The victim should continue kicking until he or she can work into a horizontal position across the top of the ice. This kicking action will not only help to propel the person onto the stronger ice, but it also will help to keep circulation moving so that the person stays warmer.

Once the victim has moved onto the ice, it is important not to stand up or kneel—body weight must remain spread out over the surface of the ice. The victim can then roll to the safety of stronger ice or to the shore. Standing or kneeling may put too much weight on a small portion of the ice and cause another breakthrough.

In aiding a person who has fallen through the ice, the rescuer must remember not to expose himself or herself to the same danger of falling through the ice. It is unwise to run to the place where the breakthrough occurred and attempt to pull out the victim. If the ice is weak enough for one person to fall through, it is not likely to be strong enough to support the rescuer. The best procedure is to offer the victim some extension item such as a rope, pole, board, stick, or other similar object. Another rescue measure is the formation of a human chain. Those forming the chain must lie down on the ice to disperse their weight. They then grasp the ankle of the person in front of them and as a group work their way forward to the spot on the ice where the victim is located. Once the victim is grasped by the lead rescuer, the human chain then slowly moves backwards.

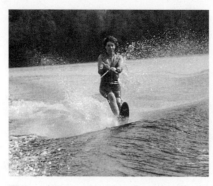 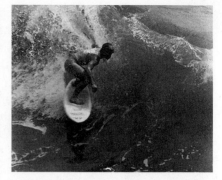

Water skiing and surfing are activities that hundreds of thousands of people take part in every year.

Once an individual has been rescued from the icy water, it is important to warm the person as quickly as possible, using coats, blankets, sweaters, and other warm pieces of clothing.

Other Water Activities

In addition to recreational boating and swimming, a number of other activities attract water enthusiasts. The more popular ones are surfing, skin diving (snorkeling), scuba diving, and water skiing.

Surfing

Surfing originated in Hawaii and has been particularly popular on the West Coast beaches of the United States. The surfer rides the crest of waves on a banana-shaped board that is nine to ten feet long and tapered at either end.

The exhilaration of this activity can be interrupted quickly if the rider is involved in a "wipeout"—that is, knocked from the board by a breaking wave. The rider may be thrown from the surfboard by losing balance or by being caught by a rough wave and thrown into the churning water. Injury is most likely to occur to the head and the neck following surfing accidents. Many times the fallen surfer may be knocked unconscious and be in need of emergency care for drowning.

Surf only where the surrounding area is designated for such activity and where emergency help is available. A safe surfing locality has no dangerous rocks and no menacing currents, tides, or undertows. No boats should be permitted in an area used by surfboard riders. It also is wise to surf with other individuals so that help could be available if one got into trouble.

Skin Diving

Below the surface of a body of water lies a world unseen except to the person prepared to dive into its depths. Beautiful fish and rock formations await individuals who have the skills and equipment necessary to swim about beneath the water's surface. For skin divers the waters' depths provide a world of beauty and silence. Skin diving, sometimes referred to as snorkeling, involves swimming about below the surface while using three pieces of equipment: a face mask, swimming fins, and snorkel.

The face mask is a rubberized goggle with unbreakable glass that can withstand the pressures of water depths. The purpose of the mask is to assist in seeing underwater and to provide protection for the eyes. The mask should cover the eyes and nose completely.

Swimming fins help propel the skin diver through the water. With swim fins the diver's hands are free for underwater exploration.

Skin divers use a snorkel for breathing while under water. The head must be near enough to the surface so that the snorkel is not submerged. Some skin divers who wish to dive deeper into the water find the snorkel a hindrance rather than a help. However, it does help to prevent fatigue as the swimmer does not have to lift his or her head each time a breath is needed.

Most accidents associated with skin diving occur when the diving area is not known. The diver should be aware of any underwater hazards. The depth of the water, the tides and current, the movement of the water, and the characteristics of the bottom and the surface should be familiar to the diver.

The skin diver must have a good sense of direction as he or she swims about. Should water enter the snorkel and get into the mouth and nose of the diver, the person must have adequate swimming skills to be able to clear both mouth and nose of the water and put the snorkel back in place while treading water. If people do not have this basic swimming skill they must not enter water that is over their head.

Scuba Diving

More hazardous than skin diving is scuba diving. This water activity is not only a recreational pursuit, but for some it is an important avocation or even vocation. Many volunteer scuba divers are called upon to dive when a body must be located after a drowning. Professional scuba divers may be asked to explore submerged objects.

Scuba diving involves swimming about under water with a self-contained source of oxygen for breathing. SCUBA means self-contained underwater breathing apparatus. Although accidents do occur, most scuba-related fatalities and/or injuries are the result of a lack of knowledge about the activity and a lack of skills needed to function properly in significant water depths.

Scuba diving places strenuous physical demands on the individual. Scuba divers must understand the various principles of physics that apply to deep water diving. For example, *caisson disease* results when the diver ascends too rapidly and nitrogen builds up in the bloodstream. This condition, potentially fatal to divers, is commonly known as the "bends."

Under normal conditions of breathing, air that is taken into the lungs contains oxygen. During exhalation oxygen, along with carbon dioxide, is given off. After inhalation there is a buildup of carbon dioxide in the lungs. Physiologically this buildup produces a subconscious urge to breathe again and normal respiration takes place. However, if pure oxygen is used, as in a closed-circuit scuba, the body may absorb more oxygen than it can use. When there has been vigorous swimming activity and prolonged deep and rapid breathing, carbon dioxide buildup is depressed and normal respiration is disrupted. This process is known as *hyperventilation*—it too, can be dangerous for divers.

The scuba diver must follow safe practices of diving. It is important always to dive with another individual. Diving should never occur when there are adverse weather and/or water conditions. No one should scuba dive unless he or she knows how to use the equipment, as well as the various principles of ascent and descent.

Scuba diving brings the recreational diver into contact with a world frequented by numerous marine animals that can cause various types of injuries. There are some one hundred species of marine animals that pose a danger to humans.[12] For example, the Portuguese Man-of-War which is found off the Florida coast gives off a toxic venom with its tentacles. The jellyfish, which is found in the waters along both the Atlantic and Pacific coasts, is the most lethal of all venomous marine animals.[13] The sting of a box jellyfish that is found in Australian waters can be fatal within one to five minutes.[14] Other examples of dangerous marine animals are sea urchins and the sea anemones.

Any person involved in scuba diving must be aware of species that are present in the waters where he or she is diving. Contact must be avoided and should contact occur the divers should attempt to stay away from the tentacles. If diving in waters where dangerous marine animals are present the diver should wear protective clothing.

If an individual is stung by a marine animal the indications will often be moderate discoloration, uncomfortable dermatitis, and throbbing pain. Treatment includes relieving the pain by treating the dermatitis and counteracting the effects of the venom.[15] Obviously these treatment modalities will necessitate medical attention.

Water Skiing

Thousands of people water ski each year. Several basic safety considerations are assumed before one water skis. People who cannot swim should never water ski. Equipment always must be checked and be in good operating condition.

The boat operator must realize the importance of careful maneuvering of the boat when pulling a skier. In addition to the boat operator, a second individual must be in the boat to monitor the person on skis. Extreme care must be taken to avoid running into the pathway of other boats or onto rocks and other obstacles in the water. Caution is paramount when pulling a person on water skis.

Water Instruction Programs

There are numerous types of water instruction programs. The American Red Cross has the most extensive programs in water safety and swimming instruction. Every year several hundred thousand persons receive instruction in the various Red Cross swimming programs. The swimming instruction program consists of several levels of swimming, from water exploration through advanced skills. The Red Cross also has a life guarding and a Water Safety Instructors' course.

There are several agencies that provide instruction for individuals operating boats. The Coast Guard Auxiliary, United States Power Squadron, and numerous state and local agencies conduct boating safety programs. On a national level the Red Cross no longer offers boating courses; however, some of the local affiliates do make instruction in boating available.

In some states it is mandated that before a young person below the age of 16 can operate a boat, he or she must have completed some type of boating safety course. These courses often are administered by an agency of the state government involved in water safety. In some states this is the state department of natural resources.

Operation Water Watch is a national program designed to prevent preschool drownings and diving injuries and deaths. This is a cooperative program of the United States Consumer Product Safety Commission and the National Spa and Pool Institute.

Canoeing instruction programs have been developed by the American Canoeing Association.

Summary

Water is an attraction for nearly everyone. There are numerous activities that occur in or near water. Basic to any water activity is the development of swimming skills.

Drowning is a major cause of fatality, particularly among young children and males between the ages of 15 and 34. The United States government has established a goal of reducing the incidences of drownings by the year 2000. To accomplish this goal it is necessary for programs to be instituted that make the public more conscious of the need for safety around water.

Drowning and injury occur in all types of water settings. Not only are ponds, rivers, lakes, and oceans localities where unintentional injury may result, but many accidents take place in home and public swimming pools.

Many different kinds of boating activities can be found on the nation's waterways. These activities involve the use of motorized boats, sailing vessels, and paddle boats. Regardless of the boat type, principles of safety and injury prevention must be followed. It is important that the operator of any boat know the various characteristics of the vessel before launching out into a body of water. The tides, currents, depth, and other essential water information also must be known for safe navigation.

A major cause of fatality and injury associated with water activities is the consumption of alcohol. Alcohol impairs many of the skills and judgments that are necessary for safe boat operation and water immersion. Measures need to be taken to alert the public to these dangers and to reduce the use of alcohol around bodies of water.

Scuba diving, skin diving, surfing, and water skiing are water activities that are very attractive to many persons. As with other water activities, it is necessary that those involved learn the unique aspects of participation. In addition, the development of skill and competence that protects against fatality and injury is important.

Discussion Questions

1. What are preventive measures that can be taken to reduce the incidences of drowning?
2. What is the danger of possessing a small degree of swimming skill?

3. Discuss the goal established by the federal government to be achieved by the year 2000 regarding drowning.
4. What is the physiological process of drowning?
5. Why is undertow a concern relating to water safety?
6. Discuss several matters that must be considered in constructing a home swimming pool.
7. Why are water slides a problem around swimming pools?
8. What measures should be considered in the safe operation of a motorboat?
9. Identify some of the procedures that need to be taken to assure safety on a boat before it is taken out on a body of water.
10. What measures do you recommend to reduce the incidence of intoxication and boat safety? Discuss.
11. Be familiar with the features and differences of each type of personal flotation device.
12. What is the effect of cold water on the immersed human body?
13. Explain emergency rescue measures when one has fallen through the ice.
14. Explain the difference between skin diving and scuba diving.
15. Identify and become familiar with some of the water instructional programs in your community.

Suggested Readings

American Red Cross. *American Red Cross National Boating Survey: A Study of Recreational Boats, Boaters, and Accidents in the United States* (Washington, DC: American Red Cross, 1991).

Auerbach, Paul S. "Stings of the Deep," *Emergency Medicine* 21, no. 12 (30 June 1989): 26–41.

Centers for Disease Control. "Alcohol Use and Aquatic Activities—United States, 1991," *Morbidity and Mortality Weekly Report* 42, no. 35 (10 September 1993): 675–82.

———. "Child Drownings and Near Drownings Associated with Swimming Pools—Maricopa County, Arizona, 1988 and 1989," *Morbidity and Mortality Weekly Report* 39, no. 26 (6 July 1990): 441–42.

———. "Drownings at U.S. Army Corps of Engineers Recreation Facilities, 1986–1990," *Morbidity and Mortality Report* 41, no. 19 (15 May 1992): 331–33.

Counts, Jan. "Canoe Safety this Summer," *Safety and Health* 141, no. 6 (June 1990): 64–65.

Gulaid, Jame A., and Richard W. Sattin. "Drownings in the United States, 1978–1984," *Morbidity and Mortality Weekly Report* 37, no. SS-1 (February 1988): 27–33.

Howland, Jonathan, and others. "A Pilot Survey of Aquatic Activities and Related Consumption of Alcohol, With Implications for Drowning," *Public Health Reports* 105, no. 4 (July–August 1990): 415.

Moler, Chris. "Drowning Prevention: A Community Affair," *Park and Recreation* 28, no. 2 (February 1993): 54–62.

Endnotes

1. National Safety Council, *Accident Facts, 1993 Edition* (Itasca, IL: National Safety Council, 1993), 4.
2. Department of Health and Human Services, *Healthy People 2000: National Health Promotion and Disease Prevention Objectives* (Washington, DC: U.S. Government Printing Office, 1991), 277.
3. Ibid.
4. Centers for Disease Control, "Position Papers from the Third National Injury Control Conference: Setting the National Agenda for Injury Control in the 1990s," *Morbidity and Mortality Weekly Report* 41, no. RR-6 (24 April 1992): 11.
5. Park E. Dietz and Susan P. Baker, "Drowning: Epidemiology and Prevention," *American Journal of Public Health* 64, no. 4 (April 1974): 311.
6. National Safety Council, *Accident Facts 1993,* 105.
7. Ibid.
8. Centers for Disease Control, "Position Papers," 11.
9. Ibid.
10. National Transportation Safety Board, *Recreational Boating Safety Study* (1993).
11. Ibid.
12. Paul S. Auerbach, "Stings of the Deep," *Emergency Medicine* 21, no. 12 (30 June 1989): 26–41.
13. Ibid.
14. William S. Hamner, "Australia's Box Jellyfish: A Killer Down Under," *National Geographic* 186, no. 2 (August, 1994): 116–130.
15. Paul S. Auerbach, "Stings of the Deep," *Emergency Medicine* 21, no. 12 (30 June 1989): 26–41.

CHAPTER 11

School Safety— Impacting People from Preschool Through the Adult Years

Chapter Outline

Introduction
Safety as Part of the Total Curriculum
  Historical Foundations
Safety Instruction
  Correlation in Specific Contexts
  The Planned Safety Curriculum
  Curriculum Packages
  Preschool Safety Instruction
  Teaching to a Plan
  Content of Safety Curricula
Safe School Environment
  The School Playground
School Bus Transportation
  Seat Belts
  The Bus Driver
  Bus Maintenance
  Bus Routes
Emergency Care
School Accident Records
Emergency Drills
  Fire Drills
  Tornado Drills
Student Involvement
School Athletics
  Personal Equipment
  Facilities
  Supervision
  Medical Care
Summary
Discussion Questions
Suggested Readings
Endnotes

Introduction

Most Americans have had some kind of formal education. In many homes, preschool activities are introduced when the child is three or four years of age. Formal schooling starts at five or six years of age and extends until individuals reach their teens. For some people, schooling continues into the adult years in college or in various kinds of professional and technical training. Today record numbers of middle-aged adults and senior citizens are taking a variety of classes to continue their education.

People study a wide range of subjects over that span of years. Basic education for coping with life's everyday activities is part of the formal school curriculum. Specific skills also are learned that enable a person to earn a living. Some learning occurs simply for the sake of broadening one's knowledge, background, and exposure. Safety education should be an important component of that schooling process.

Safety as Part of the Total Curriculum

It is doubtful that safety instruction will ever approach in status the teaching of writing, reading, mathematics, science, computers, and the social sciences. However, beginning in nursery school and extending through college, components of safety education are found in the school curriculum. What emphasis this instruction takes varies from one locality to another and from one teacher to another.

Historical Foundations

The inclusion of safety in the school curriculum had its beginnings in San Antonio, which instituted safety instruction in the schools in 1913. Similar developments followed in the cities of Detroit and Philadelphia in 1916.[1] The early programs in safety instruction usually focused on special topics. Instruction relating to fire prevention was mandated by legislation in several states. Today, in addition to requiring periodic fire drills, several states require the teaching of fire prevention.

It was not until the 1930s that more comprehensive safety courses were required by state law. One of the earliest state statutes to include all aspects of safety was passed in New York state.[2] During the 1930s programs of driver education also were introduced into school curricula.

In the years following World War II the entire school curriculum expanded. The 1960s was a time of much educational growth. During this period funds were available for experimental programs, for innovative ideas, and for the development and expansion of many school services. Teaching salaries improved, and many teachers were hired with different specialties. Federal monies were available to supply new learning centers, audiovisual rooms, language labs, and other types of educational "hardware." Some school districts funded the building of modern driving facilities for the teaching of driver and traffic safety. Driving simulators were designed for instructional use.

In recent years a variety of different movements in education have resulted in less interest in and focus on safety in the school curriculum. Voters increasingly have exercised their concerns about rising taxes and have voted against higher school funding levies. As a result many schools, particularly those in urban communities, have had to make cutbacks in various programs.

During the 1980s major concern developed throughout the nation regarding the quality of education in America. Governmental reports, commission studies, and numerous publications were released pointing out the problems in American education. Governmental and professional conferences were held to establish initiatives that would improve the quality of American education. Most of these initiatives called for increased emphasis on the basics in education: science, mathematics, communication skills, social studies, and computer literacy. Reports also called for improved teaching, greater use of educational technology, and for mandatory student testing to determine minimal success in skill acquisition. Accompanying this educational reform movement has been the concept that there are too many "frills" or nonessentials in the school curriculum. Unfortunately, among the many recommendations to improve education in the United States, safety education has never been mentioned by advocates of the educational reform movements.

Safety Instruction

In spite of the fact that safety instruction has never been considered to be a major subject for emphasis in the curriculum, many learning experiences deal with safety concepts on daily, albeit, incidental, basis. Teachers take advantage of varied situations to teach some basic concept, fact, or rule relating to safety and injury prevention. A serious motor-vehicle collision resulting in fatalities or injuries in the school community usually provides an opportunity for a discussion of traffic safety. The destruction by fire of several buildings in a downtown area presents an opportunity for study of fire prevention. The hospitalization of a classmate resulting from ingesting some toxic liquid may create much interest in learning about the dangers of poisonous substances found in and around the home.

Incidental learning experiences relating to safety can be found at any age and grade level, although this approach is used most commonly in the elementary school. It is at these younger ages that children's questions and concerns often lead to action in the classroom setting. The inquisitive nature of young children presents a natural opening for all kinds of incidental learning situations.

Correlation in Specific Contexts

Almost all safety instruction is correlated with various subject matter, as in the context of some specific academic study. This type of safety instruction takes place at both the elementary and secondary school levels. Certain subjects in the school curriculum lend themselves more naturally to the inclusion of safety concepts than do others.

The *industrial arts* or *vocational education* curriculum requires continuing attention to safety. Vocational education programs include agriculture, business/marketing, trade, and industrial educational programs. Students are prepared for employment in such fields as construction, plumbing, electrical, metal working, and auto mechanics.

The classes in which much of this education takes place require the use of a number of machines, tools, and other mechanized equipment. Students must know how to use and maintain each piece of equipment in a safe manner. Exposure to electrical current is a continuing danger in these classes. Students must be required to wear personal protective safety equipment. Eye safety is particularly important. Students must wear safety glasses and/or goggles whenever operating equipment or in any environment where it is possible that objects could become imbedded in the eyes.

Instruction must include very detailed safety measures to be taken in the operation of all equipment. While prevention of injury-causing situations is paramount in the industrial shop setting, emphasis also needs to be given to emergency care measures in case of injury. Such emphasis on learning and using safety practices will be advantageous for students as they enter the job market. They should be more productive workers if they possess a high level of concern for injury prevention.

Home economics classes present a variety of situations and learning experiences that incorporate safety concepts. The flammability of various kinds of fabrics provides opportunity for important lessons on fire and fire prevention. Certain cleaning substances have toxic properties. Students enrolled in food service programs must be taught how to use such utensils as knives, blades, blenders, and slicers in a safe manner.

The greatest number of school-related injuries in the secondary school occur in *physical education* activities. The movement involved, the competitive aspect of the games, and the aggressiveness of young people all contribute to the problem of injuries in these classes. Classes involving physical education activities should be preceded by a discussion of the kinds and possibilities of injuries associated with the given activity. Procedures designed to help reduce the incidence of injuries should be understood and practiced by the students.

Equipment used in physical education activities should not be conducive to injuries. The maintenance of equipment in safe operating order is the responsibility of the teacher. Students must be taught to use equipment and apparatus properly and at the appropriate times. Failure to do so leads to many injuries each school year.

Traditional classroom subjects also can lend themselves to the presentation of safety concepts. Take *math* class, for example: students can use statistics and data regarding injuries and fatalities in various settings to learn about safety while developing mathematical skills. In *language arts,* writing a theme or giving a speech on some safety topic would be a way to emphasize safety learning behaviors.

Many safety concepts can be incorporated into the *social studies* curriculum. Home safety, consumer safety, and community safety all provide possibilities in the context of the issues raised in government, sociology, or history units. An interesting illustration of such an approach to safety concepts was a junior high presentation on governmental regulations which focused on toy safety. Displays of toys now banned by federal regulations were shown along with a description of reasons for the ban.

Science classes provide many opportunities for presenting safety concepts. A study of electricity, its characteristics and use, should include a discussion of its potential for damage and measures needed to protect against fatal and injury-producing circumstances.

It is most common to present safety instruction in the *health education* course. A review of many state and local health education curriculum guides shows that safety is almost always a part of such instruction. However, rarely is a safety course a requirement for graduation from secondary school, and it is doubtful if such inclusion is likely in the immediate future.

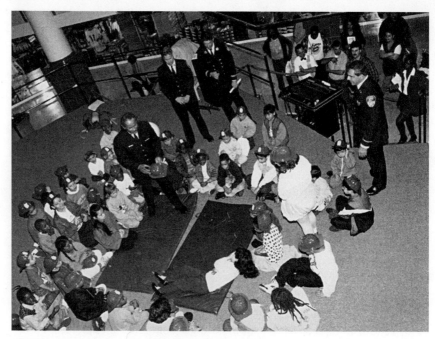

Children need to be taught to "stop-drop-roll" when their clothes catch on fire.

The Planned Safety Curriculum

The formal scheduling of a specific class in safety is most likely only at the university or college level. This course usually is a general safety class taken by students from throughout the university. Such a course may be given as an adjunct to some other program such as vocational education, agriculture, athletic training, recreation, or health/physical education.

The responsibility for curriculum development in grades K–12 is the responsibility of the local school district in most American communities. Whatever format the safety curriculum might take can vary significantly from one school system to another. Hence, it is important to analyze the specific safety curriculum to determine if the program is designed to meet the specific needs of children living in the particular community served by the school.

A number of community agencies and organizations provide safety instructional programs for use in the school. Usually these activities focus on a special component of injury prevention. In some instances these efforts are designed to coincide with special dates or weeks of national or local emphasis.

Since the early 1920s the National Fire Prevention Association has proclaimed a week in October to be Fire Prevention Week. The week selected extends from Sunday through Saturday of the week that includes October 9, the anniversary of the great fire in Chicago in 1872. During this week personnel from the local fire department usually come to the schools to provide instruction and demonstrations for the children. A fire drill is often scheduled at school sometime during National Fire Prevention Week.

Another special occasion is National Farm Safety Week, jointly sponsored by the National Safety Council and the U.S. Department of Agriculture. A different accident problem is highlighted each year. Educational programs, posters, and public radio and television spots are presented to emphasize safety in rural localities.

In many communities personnel from the local police department can be counted on to provide a class on some aspect of safe living. The session varies according to the age level of the students. It may include a class on pedestrian safety or procedures to use walking to and from school for younger children. In the spring the police department may conduct a bicycle roundup. The students bring their bicycles to school, have them checked for safe operation, and then often participate in a competitive "rodeo."

Police officers feel that such exposure in a teaching capacity in the school safety program does more than impart safety facts. They also see the public relations value in such activity. It is hoped that a school-aged child will view the police officer as a friend and as a person to count on for help and assistance in the community rather than only as a law enforcement officer.

Curriculum Packages

There are many safety curriculum packages that have been designed by various government and voluntary safety and health organizations. These vary in content and approach, as well as in appropriateness for different ages and grade levels. Some are more inclusive than others.

The Consumer Product Safety Commission has developed an elementary safety program designed to teach children the importance of using seat belts and to educate older children in product safety.[3] The primary grades (K–3) curriculum is entitled *A Safer Way For Everyday*. This six-lesson program focuses on the need to use seat belts while riding in automobiles. Learning activity sheets are available for each of the six lessons. Each learning activity begins with vocabulary listing of words used in the particular lesson that might be unfamiliar to the children. Parental support and involvement is encouraged in this program with the inclusion of a Parent's Night.

The Consumer Product Safety Commission program for grades 3 through 6 is entitled *It's No Accident*. This curriculum is designed to teach safety habits and practices that will reduce product-related injuries. Prevention of injury, personal control, and responsibility are emphasized in the different learning experiences. There are eight units included in this program:

1. General overview of consumer product safety
2. Home fire safety
3. Playground safety
4. Bicycle, roller skating, skateboard safety
5. Poison prevention
6. Toy safety
7. Holiday safety
8. Electrical safety

A teacher's resource file is included with this program, offering suggested classroom questions and individual activities for use in each grade level. Stories and puzzles to accompany the learning experiences are available. The learning objectives are stated in terms of specific competencies for each of the eight units.

Several curriculum programs are available from the American Red Cross that can be included in a school safety instructional program.[4] A bicycle safety course is available for use in all elementary grades (grades 1 through 6). Another elementary (grade 1 through 6) program on home safety is designed to help children become aware of the many dangers around the home and how to prevent injury.

The Red Cross has developed a course on baby-sitting directed toward fifth and sixth grade children. The course is designed to help adolescents be more effective baby-sitters. Overall safety concepts are included in this program. The students are taught how to cope with emergencies and illnesses that might arise while taking care of younger children. They are taught how to feed, play with, and care for youngsters. Upon completion of this program the Red Cross issues a certificate signifying that the recipient has completed this course. This certification provides evidence to parents that the adolescent they have engaged to baby-sit with their children has received some useful instruction.

Preschool Safety Instruction

It is during the preschool years of a child's life that safety attitudes develop. The *Safety Town Program* is an educational series designed specifically to teach preschoolers about safety.[5] The program instills an awareness of the importance of safety in all aspects of life.

The major focus of the Safety Town Program is traffic safety. Playground safety, toy and home safety, and water safety also receive attention.

Participatory learning is the major teaching technique. Children are placed in simulated situations, and a miniature town (Safety Town) is constructed, providing opportunities to teach a variety of skills. The teaching approach is based on research about the mental and physical abilities of preschoolers. The two-week program is held primarily during the summer.

The National Safety Town Center which has developed this program usually works with local community and civic organizations in conducting the activities. The Center provides the materials; parental involvement is also included.

Teaching to a Plan

No one denies the value of safety education programs and curriculum materials. All have as their goal improved safety and well-being for school-aged children. However, the hit-or-miss approach currently applied to safety curriculum planning in many school districts must be questioned. Such a scattered focus precludes progressive presentation of safety information. Disassociated programming probably continues because it seems convenient to the teacher or school administrator. Given the expense and time involved in planning and presenting material, the responsibility for developing safety instruction tends to fall to agencies or organizations concerned with safety issues, not to the school district.

However, school administrators and safety instructors need to work for a comprehensive school safety curriculum based on the needs and interests of students. Curriculum planning must identify specific competencies and performance skills for the various grade levels. Once these are clear, teaching strategies can be designed to provide worthwhile learning activities in safety education. If the services of a community agency or organization are required to fill the need for specific instruction, they should be used. However, the curriculum must not be regulated by the individualized interests of outside groups.

Content of Safety Curricula

The content to be taught in a safety lesson varies. It is not possible, nor is it desirable, to teach the same information in all school systems at the same level. Students' needs and interests vary from one location to another. The child who lives on the farm has different needs from the child living in the urban inner city. To become familiar with what might be included in the school safety curriculum, it is useful to examine several curriculum guides developed by state departments of education. Also, many local districts have curriculum materials outlined and available for examination.

Differences of opinion among safety educators exist as to what should be taught in the school safety program. For example, traditionally it has been taught that a pedestrian must cross a street at the intersection. Many people can remember learning such a safety rule as a youngster—cross only at the corner. In reality, however, many children, as well as adults, cross streets in midblock. Therefore, some would suggest that children should be taught safe measures for crossing a street when not at an intersection. Others believe that to instruct school children to cross at midblock is actually teaching them to perform an illegal act since it may be against the law to jaywalk. So the debate continues. Should we emphasize obeying the law and ignore the reality of the situation—that people will cross streets at places other than the intersections? Or should we teach children to cross streets safely at any point in the block?

It seems that the objective of safety education is to help people cope with the reality of life. To learn a rule and ignore *what is* misses the real need of the students. It seems important that safety be taught *conceptually.* Safety concepts that may apply to a variety of settings must be the focus of the teaching-learning situation. Isolated situations or freak examples must never be central to teaching. Then most issues raised in debates about safety education can be resolved.

Safe School Environment

Not only should there be instruction within the school curriculum concerning safety, but the school environment within which a child spends a significant portion of each day must be as free as possible from injury-causing agents and conditions. There is a clear expectation that schools will provide a safe environment for every person who comes to the school: students, parents, and community citizens.

Children are sent to school by their parents with the understanding that their well-being will not be endangered while in the classroom.

The mandatory nature of school attendance from about age seven until fifteen or sixteen implies institutional responsibility for children's safety and well-being.

School buildings must be constructed so that as few potential hazards as possible are present. This necessitates a focus on student safety during the planning and designing of new school buildings. The initial planning of a school building must take into consideration the site location. Schools, if at all possible, should be located away from busy streets and roads. This is difficult to accomplish in most urban settings.

The layout of play areas, walks, and recreational facilities on the school grounds should protect against overlap of activities that can result in injuries. The elementary school play area should not be located next to the area in which the junior high school students are playing baseball, for example. Natural structures such as trees and bushes should not be on playgrounds and athletic fields. Water drainage ditches should not be located in such school areas.

All school buildings need to be maintained in good repair. This is particularly important in older schools. Personnel must be employed and funds allocated for building maintenance and repair. In some school districts it has been necessary to reduce the amount of building maintenance and repair for economic reasons. As school administrators are forced to make operating cutbacks due to reduced school funding and rising operational costs, badly needed building repairs are often postponed. The taxpayer is much more likely to support funding for a school science, reading, or special education program than for badly needed school maintenance or repairs.

Potential hazards within the school building and on school grounds must be identified and then eliminated. Every school employee—whether a teacher, administrator, or staff member—must report any potentially dangerous condition observed about the school to the proper authority.

The responsibility also necessitates maintaining any equipment that the students use in safe and functional condition. Within every school there are numerous kinds of equipment that the children use daily. It is the responsibility of school personnel to supervise the use of all equipment. When not in use, equipment should be stored in a location where there is the least possibility for student access. Whenever any type of equipment is used, students should be instructed in its safe use prior to participation. Periodically after that initial instruction, a review of safety regulations should be presented as part of the class instructional experience.

The School Playground

Most schools, particularly elementary schools, have a playground area in which children participate in a number of activities before and after the school day; in addition such grounds provide a place for many activities during the school day. Thousands of injuries occur each school year on the playground. The most common playground injuries result from falls. Some 60 to 70 percent of playground-related injuries are caused when children fall from equipment.

A number of factors contribute to student injuries. One major factor—affecting the number and severity of injuries—relates to the type of surface on which the equipment is located. Many school playgrounds have asphalt, concrete, or packed-earth surfaces. These provide no injury protection and are unsuitable for use on playgrounds.

More resilient surface materials should be used on school playgrounds. Sand, wood chips, protective mats, and shredded tires provide more protection from injury, reduce the severity of injuries, and are recommended for use on playgrounds by the Consumer Product Safety Commission. However, these materials all require continuous maintenance and are more expensive than concrete or asphalt.

Other problems are associated with safety on playgrounds. Proper supervision and maintenance are very important. Injuries often result from defects in the construction, wear, and design of equipment. Children must be instructed in proper use of all playground equipment on the school grounds.

Planning and construction of a school playground must include considerations for student safety. For example, swings should be in place with seats of rubber, nylon, canvas, or plastic, not wood, aluminum, or metal. Well-planned playgrounds should provide a wide variety of play situations where children can run, swing, climb, slide, push, and pull in creative play experiences. Adequate space between each piece of equipment is important.

A need exists for the development of standards for school playgrounds. Guidelines have been recommended by the American Academy of Pediatrics as well as the National Recreation and Parks Association. These guidelines need to be studied by school administrators and implemented for improved safety on school playgrounds.

School Bus Transportation

The school bus is probably the most common public motor vehicle found in nearly every American community. School buses come in a variety of sizes, but universally they are yellow with black lettering on

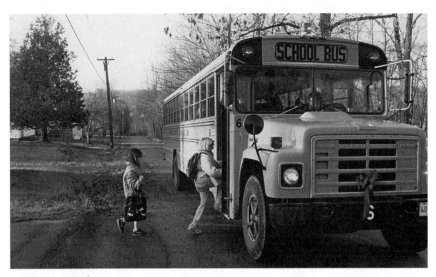

Every school day, as many as 22 million children ride a bus to school. Color and markings on school buses are standardized throughout the United States.

the sides. The words School Bus appear in several places on the exterior along with the name of the school district. Federal law requires that the words School Bus appear both on the front and the rear of the bus. It is also required that school buses be yellow and have bumpers painted with a glossy black color. School buses must have signal lights as well as a mirror system that enables the driver to see each side of the bus. This provides better control and visibility as the children are getting on the bus and after they have disembarked. This requirement is particularly important in that over 80 percent of fatalities relating to school buses occur to pupils as pedestrians, either approaching or leaving a loading zone.

Except for some children living in urban areas or residing very close to their individual school buildings, most youngsters ride a school bus at some point during their school days. It is estimated that some 22 million children ride to school on school buses each day of the school year. More than 380,000 buses are operated by public and private school systems. Some 4.4 billion miles are covered each year by school buses.[6]

With this heavy volume of bus traffic, there are going to be injuries involving school bus collisions. Approximately 8,300 children were injured in a recent year from accidents involving school buses. A total of 110 individuals were killed during one recent year in school bus accidents; 35 of these were children. Ten of these fatalities involved passengers on school buses and the remainder either occurred to children approaching or leaving a school bus loading zone.[7] Many of the fatalities occur when motorists illegally pass a standing school bus.

Considering the numbers of children riding school buses each day, it is a wonder that the incidences of injury and fatality are as low as they are. However, when considering the nature of those riding the school bus, young children with a future ahead of them, school systems cannot be too careful in taking steps to improve the safety of school bus transportation.

For this reason, research and development needs to be continued to provide safer school buses. Improvements through the engineering research and development should make for safer vehicles. For example, measures have been implemented to eliminate blind spots in front of the bus. Also, there is need for backing-up alarm systems to alert children when the bus is to be operated in reverse. New strobe light systems help to make bus visibility more effective in fog and darkness. In some instances outside address systems are used where the driver can communicate with the students in the loading zone. Different states mandate different safety systems.

Seat Belts

There has been much discussion and debate as to whether seat belts should be required on school buses. Since 1977 with the passage of the Highway Safety Act, the National Highway Traffic and Safety Agency has required that every person riding a school bus must be provided with a seat in which to sit. These seats must be close enough together so that a child will not be thrown about upon impact. It is felt that such construction of the bus will compartmentalize the occupants and keep them from being thrown about.

However, many feel that this is inadequate. Supporters of lap belts in school buses emphasize that padded backs of seats give little protection and are of little help if the bus should turn over in a collision or if the bus is struck from the side. It is also felt that requiring the students on school buses to use the belts would serve an educational role. The children would learn to fasten the belt upon sitting in the seat as he or she should do upon entering an automobile. The need for lap belts in school buses has been endorsed by many different groups, such as the American College of Surgeons and the American College of Emergency Physicians. The National Coalition for Seat Belts in School Buses was formed in 1984 to support actions to mandate seat belt use in school buses.

On the other hand, the National Transportation Safety Administration and the National School Transportation Association are not supporters of seat belt use in school buses. Major opposition to mandating lap belts on school buses tends to focus on the cost of equipping older buses. Also, opponents question whether bus drivers are in a position to carry out the responsibility to assure that all children are properly seated with the belts properly in place.

In 1989 a report of the National Transportation Safety Board concluded that requiring seat belts on school buses is of minimal value. It would be of more value to raise the minimum height of seat backs and increase efforts to provide safer loading zones. This report also pointed out the need for better selection and training of bus drivers.

The NTSB report noted that all buses manufactured before April 1, 1977 should be replaced. Though not legally binding, the National Transportation Safety Board recommendations included several safety improvements for school buses:

1. reinforcement of roof and body joints on the bus structure
2. inclusion of pop-out windows
3. use of fire retardant seat covers
4. construction of more accessible exit doors
5. construction of rupture-proof fuel tanks

The report also suggested that schools should conduct school bus evacuation drills and stated that children should be instructed on how to get on and off the bus in a safe manner.

The Bus Driver

School bus drivers must be selected, trained, and supervised with an eye toward reducing fatalities and injuries. There is much more to being an effective and safe school bus driver than simply being able to maneuver the vehicle along the streets and roads of a community.

School bus drivers should know the basic mechanics of bus operation. They also should see that the bus is maintained in a clean condition and have responsibility for explaining to the children and enforcing the various safety rules and regulations.

There is little doubt that the driver plays an important role in the lives of the school children. This person can be a friendly, safety-oriented person, liked and respected by the children. Or the individual may give little consideration to the children except that which is demanded by the law. School bus drivers should recognize their role as part of the total school safety experience of the children.

The selection procedures and the training of school bus drivers varies from one school district to another. Some states do not require school bus driver training. Some states require that before an individual can serve as a school bus driver a physical examination is required. Though it is not likely, it would seem logical to suggest that some type of federal regulatory mandates be established for training and minimum qualifications of school bus drivers.

All bus drivers should receive in-service instruction concerning their tasks and responsibilities. Drivers should be between 25 and 60 years of age, since it is questionable that younger or older individuals should be given the responsibility of fifty or more children.

Not only should the school bus driver be able to drive and handle the vehicle in a safe manner, but the individual also has responsibility for maintaining control of the children riding on the bus. Certain safe riding rules must be developed by the school administration; the children should be instructed regarding these regulations; and then the rules should be enforced.

Instruction regarding school bus safety should be part of the school curriculum. Children who ride school buses should receive ongoing instruction concerning safe riding practices. They must be informed where to stand alongside the street or road until the bus arrives and also be knowledgeable about procedures to follow when disembarking from a bus.

Children should be expected to remain seated at all times while riding a school bus. They should also know what measures and rules to follow in case of an emergency. Conducting emergency evacuation drills can be very useful. Children should not only know the various rules to be followed while riding the bus, but they also should be expected to obey the instructions of the school bus driver. While riding the bus, the driver should have the authority to maintain control of all children. The driver should explain the rules and then make sure that they are enforced.

Bus Maintenance

An important component in operating a school bus program is ensuring that the vehicles are maintained in safe operating condition. This means that all school districts must conduct an ongoing program of preventive maintenance. Extensive vehicle inspection should be conducted twice a year. Each day before starting, the individual driver should perform an inspection of the bus. It is impossible to be too careful in the maintenance and inspection of school buses used in transporting the children.

Bus Routes

After careful review and planning, the school district should establish school bus routes. If possible, loading and unloading zones should not be located on heavily traveled roads and streets. Boarding locations should be convenient for each child; however, it is not necessary that each child be picked up at his or her own home. Children can be expected to walk a reasonable distance to meet the school bus.

A universal traffic safety rule is that any motor vehicle must not pass a school bus that is stopped for the purpose of taking on or discharging pupils. The motor vehicle should not proceed until the red warning signals are turned off. In several instances local highway regulations do not require oncoming traffic to stop for a school bus where there is a multiple-lane roadway with a highway divider. However, unless one is sure of the local law, it is wise to come to a halt when approaching a stopped school bus. The operator of the motor vehicle should not move forward until the school bus has begun to move or the school bus driver has signaled that it is safe for the traffic behind the vehicle to pass.

Unfortunately, several fatalities and injuries occur each year resulting from motorists illegally passing a stopped school bus. In order to reduce these actions of negligent drivers, laws are needed to enforce stricter penalties and to prosecute drivers who pass school buses that are loading and unloading students. Some safety leaders believe it would be legally acceptable to permit reports from witnesses of license numbers of vehicles which fail to stop for school buses.

Emergency Care

Regardless of the efforts made to protect against injury in the school setting, thousands of injuries occur annually. For this reason, effective measures must be established to render emergency care to children during the school day.

When a child becomes sick or is injured while at school, the best of care should be provided. This is not always the case. Many times emergency care facilities within the school are lacking. Often the teacher refuses to provide the care needed for fear of legal entanglements. Other reasons for not providing effective emergency care include: (1) inadequate training or skill on the part of the teacher or school supervisor, (2) administrative regulations prohibiting such assistance except in "life-threatening" situations, and (3) poor interaction between the schools and community agencies involved in the provision of emergency services.

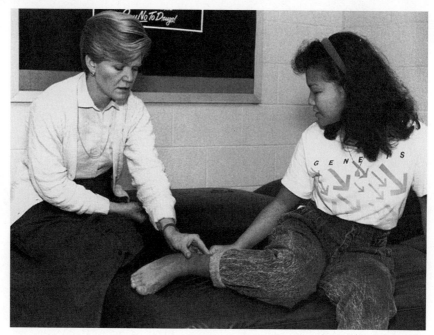

School personnel need to be able to render appropriate emergency care to sick or injured children at school.

Two basic components must be taken into account in rendering emergency aid to the school child. The first deals with providing emergency aid at the scene of the injury—the school. The second deals with obtaining the needed follow-up care and medical treatment for the sick or injured child, which of necessity will involve various community safety services.

At the scene of the injury there appears to be little question that the responsible teacher or other school personnel have a mandate to render immediate emergency care. The courts have found that failure to render aid constitutes negligent behavior on the part of the teacher. This means when such incidents occur as bleeding, ingestion of some poisonous substance, burns, possible fractures, respiration stoppage, or similar emergencies, the school cannot take a "hands-off" position. Someone must take action to assist the child. It must be clear what responsibilities and duties the teachers have at this time.

Many schools designate the school nurse or the physical education teacher to provide needed care. In some schools the school secretary cares for the sick or injured child. What happens if the nurse is in another building when an injury occurs? Why should the physical education teacher be singled out to render emergency care to students in other classes? These kinds of policies and procedures are in need of change. All school personnel should be required to possess the skills necessary for rendering basic emergency care.

Provision for giving first aid treatment to children does not occur in some schools except in life-threatening situations. Usually a child is kept in an emergency room or the nurse's room and the parents are called when injury occurs. The parents then are expected to come to the school and see that proper care is rendered. The question raised by such a policy is, What is a life-threatening situation? Who makes that determination? Every injury, regardless of its magnitude, should be cared for as soon as possible.

There should be an emergency medical form on file for each child in every school which authorizes the school to take certain actions when needed. The physician to be contacted in case of an emergency should be identified. Parents, another relative, or neighbor should indicate where they can be reached throughout the day. Notification has become an increasingly difficult issue as more mothers work outside the home during the school day; there is no one at home for the school to contact in case of an injury.

When an injured child must be taken to the emergency room of a hospital from the school, the hospital often will not administer the needed care until the parents or legal guardians have signed on behalf of their child. Certainly hospitals have legitimate liability reasons for such regulations. Yet it is difficult to understand why a child should have to wait in an emergency room, often experiencing pain and discomfort, and not be treated until some kind of permission is given by the parent.

One reason for the conflict and difference of opinion over the actions to be taken at school regarding the sick and the injured is the difference in terminology used by various people. In one case, for example, an elementary school principal presenting school policy at a new teacher orientation meeting states: "You are not to render any first aid." In pursuing this concept with the principal, it was acknowledged that any bleeding should be stopped, any cuts and scratches cared for, all burns attended to, and so on. Further questioning revealed that what was prohibited was the issuing of medicines. For instance, it was forbidden to give a child an aspirin. The concept of emergency care to this principal did not focus on the emergency injury-causing situation, but rather on medical care.

Considering the complexity of rendering emergency care to school children, every school board must develop written policies for comprehensive emergency care. Every teacher, school employee, parent, and child should know exactly what measures will be taken in case of an accident while at school. Such policies should be developed after consultation with local school administrative authorities, medical personnel, legal specialists, and parents. Once these policies are agreed upon, they should be made available in writing to all concerned parties. Such regulations will assure that school children receive proper, efficient, and immediate care when injured or a child becomes ill while at school.

School Accident Records

Records of accidents that occur in conjunction with school activities need to be maintained by the schools. There are many different kinds of accident report forms with varying amounts of information. Some school districts develop their own forms. Others use forms developed for use by the state. The National Safety Council has developed a form that is useful for school districts. No matter how the form is developed, description of the accident and the injuries sustained by students should be noted, the emergency care performed at the time of the incident should be recorded, and the personnel in charge of the activity or the area in which the incident occurred should be indicated. The individual in charge at the time of the occurrence should complete the report form.

Policy needs to be established as to which kinds of accidents are to be reported and which are not. Minor bruises, bumps, and scratches sustained around the building or on the playground probably do not need to be reported. However, any occurrence necessitating medical care should be reported. Also if the student misses at least a half day of school because of the injury, an accident report should be filed.

One important reason for insisting on accident report forms is the potential for legal or medical insurance involvement. If a future lawsuit is filed, the accurate recording of events and actions at the time would be useful.

Accident reports also give the school administration data as to the location and causes of injury-related incidents throughout the school building and on the school grounds. Locations at which injuries occur most commonly can be noted. The types of accidents and related injuries can be identified. When the data reveal an abnormal number of occurrences in a certain location in or around the school, active steps can be taken to reduce or eliminate the specific hazards.

Emergency Drills

Students in school should be prepared to take prearranged protective actions in case of fire or natural disaster. This necessitates conducting practice drills throughout the school year so that every student will be able to function safely in times of emergency.

Fire Drills

Every person who has attended school, from nursery school through college, has experienced a fire drill. To the elementary school child the fire drill is exciting. However, for the high school and college student the practice of vacating a school building for a fire drill has become commonplace. In fact the college student may stay in his or her room rather than leave the building or may remain in a remote library carrel during a fire drill. This nonchalant attitude toward the emergency drill could at some time result in personal disaster.

Fire drills are required on a regular basis in schools. The specific times and regularity vary from one state to another and from one school district to another. It is important that whenever they are conducted, fire drills are treated as an effective learning activity and not just an exercise to be carried out to fulfill some law.

Students must be familiar with primary, as well as secondary, exit routes to the outside from locations within the school building. They need to know where to assemble once outside the building. All students and other personnel in the building should be accounted for once they have left the school building.

Rarely are measures designed to simulate realism in a fire drill. What would happen if the stairway that the students were to use as the primary route was on fire? How would the students react if sirens and flashing fire engine lights were present at the school during the drill? Would panic occur if simulated smoke were present? School fire drills should incorporate measures of realism. For example, blocking one doorway and prohibiting students from using it would require immediate change to an alternate exit. Using a smoke bomb in one hallway can add realism. Although panic and disorderly exit might result, it would be much better to experience such actions when it is a drill rather than when there is a fire.

Fire drills should be conducted throughout the school year, not just in the early fall and late spring when the weather is nice and children do not have to put on their heavy coats and boots in cold weather locations. It is also unwise to announce a fire drill in advance. It is not unusual to have the younger children be given instruction to get their coats and boots on several minutes before dismissal time because of a fire drill. This kind of action does little to prepare the children for the reality of the situation in case of fire.

Tornado Drills

In several parts of the country tornado drills are conducted as part of the school safety program. Children should be instructed to exit those rooms having windows that could be blown out by the tornado winds. They should put their faces down and cover their heads with their hands. Those areas that provide the greatest amount of shelter for children should be selected. Basement locations are probably the safest; hallways or rooms without windows are also acceptable. Larger rooms such as gymnasiums and auditoriums should be avoided because they lack strong structural supports. The wind of a tornado can blow off a roof and the surrounding walls may collapse.

The warning signals unique to a tornado drill must be identified. The children must know the difference between a tornado drill warning and some other emergency warning, such as a fire drill. Misunderstanding of the specific warning signal could be tragic. In the case of a fire drill the children should be taught to leave the building and go to safety outdoors. In the case of a tornado the last thing that should happen is for the students to be instructed to go outside with the tornado winds approaching the locality of the school building.

Student Involvement

School children of all ages should be encouraged to improve the safety environment of their school buildings. Often it has been found that the establishment of certain safety rules are of little value because the students have not internalized the importance of the matter. This is particularly true for secondary school and college students.

Students should be encouraged to recognize potentially dangerous conditions at school and recommend ways in which to reduce the problem. One successful resolution occurred in a high school in which several injuries had occurred on a particular stairway. There clearly were several crosscurrents of traffic on the stairs as students moved from one class to another. The school administrator knew that to impose a certain flow pattern would be of little value as the students would not adhere to it and would view such a mandate negatively.

The issue was examined by a group of senior students as a class project in a course on civic and community government. The students gathered data indicating that this particular hallway/stairway had the greatest potential for injury occurring in the school. Through a process of group dynamics in the classroom, a recommendation for traffic flow was presented to the school administration by these students. Interestingly, the plan was little different from what the faculty and administration had recommended. However, because students internalized and identified with the issues, an effective solution was reached. Any school, at any grade level, should encourage student involvement in identifying hazards in and around the school setting. Not only should hazards be noted, but solutions should be designed and implemented. Such practices will begin to provide students with decision-making skills that will have application in the future for them as adults.

School Athletics

Sports and athletic programs are extremely important in schools throughout the United States. Collectively, hundreds of thousands of hours and participants are involved in various school athletic activities. Some of these events play major roles in their communities with thousands of people attending the contests, such as football games in Texas, Florida, and Ohio schools, or basketball in the schools of Indiana. Many others involve participation with little public interest or fanfare, such as wrestling, cross-country running, or bowling.

Regardless of the level of competition, however, from grades seven through college more than half of all school-related injuries occur in physical education activities, intramural and interscholastic sporting events. This is true for both boys and girls.

Athletic and sporting competition lend themselves to potential for collisions, falls, and accompanying injuries. Yet few people are willing to suggest that such activities be eliminated from the schools. As a matter of fact, in some communities, when it has become necessary for economic reasons to consider reducing, or eliminating, the interscholastic sports program, interested agencies or businesses have donated substantial funds to continue athletics. In many school districts parents are being asked to provide payment to the schools so that their children can participate in a sports program. The pressure from the community to maintain strong athletic programs is evident. There is little question that such activities play a valuable role in American culture and society. Therefore, it is necessary to consider ways in which to ensure as safe an environment as possible for those students involved in athletics.

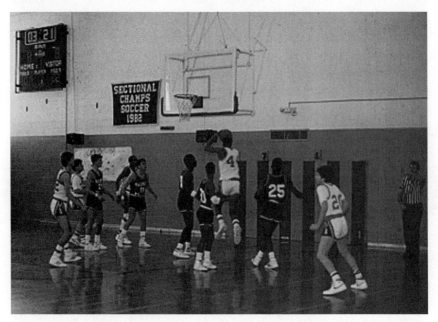

Interscholastic athletics are important in the schools of communities throughout the United States. Part of the practice and preparation in all sports should be the introduction of measures designed to reduce the likelihood of injury.

Personal Equipment

Most athletic activities make use of some kind of equipment. In many sports, equipment worn by the participant is important for protecting against injury. In football this means wearing helmets and shoulder and hip pads. In softball and baseball it means wearing a batting helmet. Shoes are important in all sports. It is important to select shoes that provide protection against foot and ankle injuries. All personal equipment should be designed to provide as much protection from injury as possible. It should fit properly and should be required for practice as well as for the game.

It is wise to spend money for the best equipment available. Use of cheaper, substandard equipment may result in injuries that in the long run are more costly than the outlay for the more expensive equipment would have been.

Facilities

Sports activities are conducted in a variety of different locations. Football, soccer, and field hockey are played on grass or dirt surfaces. Many colleges and some high schools now use artificial turf. Differences of opinion exist over whether the artificial surfaces are safer than natural grass. Ankle injuries seem to be less frequent on the artificial surfaces; however, bruises and fractures are more common.

Indoor athletic activities are carried out on wooden or similar hard surfaces that must be maintained so that injury does not occur. Protective mats need to be in place to provide some protection in such activities as basketball, volleyball, and wrestling. Maintenance of mats and floors needs to provide for safety of the participants.

Many injuries occur when players collide with an object along the sidelines, such as spectator seats, a light post, or a wall. Measures should be taken when constructing playing facilities to eliminate such obstacles. Any potentially dangerous structure must be well padded. Regardless of location, care must be taken to keep hazardous objects, such as glass, stones, and other debris away from the playing areas.

Supervision

Injuries resulting from athletic participation can be reduced by careful, continuous supervision. The degree of direct supervision of an activity relates to the age and level of skill of the students involved. Younger children require the closest supervision. However, teachers, coaches, and other school personnel have responsibility for supervision regardless of the age and grade level.

Injury results in some instances because the participants are improperly matched by size, strength, maturity, and skill. This is most common in physical education classes and in intramural sports activities. The practice of classifying youngsters by age or grade level is not always acceptable when considering safety; at any given age, size or skill groups vary greatly.

Any individual participating in competitive interscholastic athletics should be in proper physical condition for the selected activity. High school athletic associations in most states require a period of conditioning before practice can begin for sports such as football, basketball, and soccer. Before body contact is permitted, a required length of time must be devoted to conditioning. Conditioning is specific to the particular sport, and every teacher and coach responsible for an athletic activity should know how to condition their particular participants. They should see that such conditioning activities take place and that no one is permitted to participate who fails to meet certain levels of physical conditioning. Such measures will help to reduce injury.

Medical Care

Most participants in interscholastic athletics must have a preseason physical examination before being permitted to play on a team. How effective and comprehensive these measures are must be questioned. Too often physical examinations consist of a quick check of the heart and lungs by a physician with little else being considered. Rarely is the child's body type, a complete medical history, blood and urinalysis, and the specific kind of athletic participation considered.

Certain physical conditions may prevent an individual from participating in one sport, yet the child is able to take part in another activity. Rarely are athletic physical examinations sport specific. An identified handicap should not necessarily disqualify one from total physical involvement. There needs to be greater communication between physicians and those involved in athletics so that if a physical handicap is noted, measures can be taken to get the student into other activities if appropriate.

Some educational and medical personnel have suggested that national standards should be established for physical examinations for athletic participation. This is important since there are variations in requirements for physicals between states and in many instances between school districts. For example, in some states it is only necessary for the student to provide a certificate signed by the personal physician indicating that the individual is able to participate in athletics. In other states standardized forms have been prepared in which background information must be provided about the family medical history.

It seems logical to require that every person participating in intramural sports as well as in physical education classes have a physical examination. The practice of allowing students who for physical reasons cannot play interschool basketball or some other sport to then play intramural sports is open to question.

The school district has the responsibility for rendering assistance to participants who become injured during athletic practice or competition. Most colleges and universities and some high schools have athletic trainers. The National Athletic Trainers Association has been instrumental in upgrading the training and certification of personnel to serve schools as athletic trainers. As a result, certification is now required for athletic trainers in some states. Unfortunately, such trainers are generally not available for what is considered to be the minor sports, for practices, and for intramural activities.

Lack of available personnel to serve as trainers during practice and at many games to care for the injured is a significant problem. Coaches should not be expected to render emergency care to an injured participant. It is a coach's responsibility to continue coaching and working with the team. He or she cannot be expected to give time and the needed attention to an injured athlete. This matter needs the attention of the coaches and the school administration.

Summary

For many years safety has been included as part of the total school program. Yet safety instruction has never been considered a major subject in the educational curriculum. A number of different approaches and learning strategies are used for teaching safety and injury prevention concepts. Whatever teaching strategies are used, they must contribute to the overall goal of safety instruction, which is positive safety behavior.

The school setting in which a child spends several hours each school day must be as free of hazards as possible. Many measures need to be taken to assure a safe school setting. School buildings must be maintained and supervision of children planned in order to protect against situations which result in injury to students. School playgrounds should be designed to provide as safe an environment as possible.

Each day thousands of children are transported to school on school buses. Maintenance of buses, employment of responsible school bus drivers, and several other factors are important in providing the safe operation of school buses.

All school personnel should be expected to be able to render emergency care when a child is injured or becomes sick while at school. Measures must be taken to obtain the needed care for a child in these circumstances. Written records should be kept of any accident resulting in school absence of at least one-half day or any injury requiring medical attention.

Measures should be taken to teach students how to react in time of an emergency. Realism should be built into fire drills and drills designed to protect against other calamities.

Discussion Questions

1. Do you believe that safety instruction in the school curriculum should be considered to be a major subject for study? Explain your answer.
2. Identify some of the early school safety programs in the nation.
3. Discuss some of the ways in which safety concepts are taught in the schools.

4. How are safety concepts correlated with various subjects in the school curriculum?
5. Give examples of safety instructional packages provided by outside community agencies.
6. Why are school personnel responsible for the safety of children while at school?
7. Do you support requiring that seat belts be placed on all school buses? Why or why not?
8. Discuss the conclusions reached by the National Transportation Safety Board in 1989 regarding safety belts on school buses.
9. Do you agree that every school teacher should be expected to render emergency care to injured or sick children? Why or why not?
10. Identify some concerns about the construction and organization of a school playground.
11. What are several purposes served by keeping school accident records?
12. Would you encourage that a fire simulation be used during a school fire drill? Give reasons for your answer.
13. Identify other types of emergencies that demand the need for school drills.
14. What are procedural differences between a fire drill and a tornado drill?
15. Discuss measures that can be taken to reduce the likelihood of injury among participants in school sports programs.
16. Should every school have an athletic trainer? Discuss your answer.

Suggested Readings

Bass, Joel L., Kishor A. Mehta, and Bonnie M. Eppes. "What School Children Need to Learn About Injury Prevention," *Public Health Reports* 104, no. 4 (July–August 1989): 385–88.

Centers for Disease Control. "Playground-Related Injuries in Preschool-Aged Children—United States, 1983–1987," *Morbidity and Mortality Weekly Report* 37, no. 41 (21 October 1988): 629–32.

———. "Football-Related Spinal Cord Injuries Among High School Players—Louisiana, 1989," *Morbidity and Mortality Weekly Report* 39, no. 34 (31 August 1990): 586–87.

Frederick, Roxanne A., and David M. White. "Safety and First Aid Behavioral Intentions of Supervised and Unsupervised Third Grade Students," *Journal of School Health* 59, no. 4 (April 1989): 146–48.

Goldberg, Barry, and others. "Injuries in Youth Football," *Pediatrics* 80, no. 2 (February 1988): 255–61.

Kerr, Dianne Lynne. "School Bus Safety: Focus on the Danger Zone," *Journal of School Health* 57, no. 6 (August 1987): 237–39.

Lee, E. Juanita, and Joan M. Jacobson. "Accident Reports: Survey of High School Injuries," *Pediatric Nursing* 13, no. 3 (May–June 1987): 151–54.

Micheli, Lyle J. "Children and Sports," *Newsweek* (29 October 1990): 12.

Wilson, Carol Jo. "Playground Safety," *School Nurse* (October 1990): 36–39.

Endnotes

1. Carl Willgoose, *Health Teaching in Secondary Schools* (Philadelphia: W. B. Saunders, 1977), 307.
2. Richard K. Means, *Historical Perspectives on School Health,* (Thorofare, J.J.: Slack, 1975), 39.
3. U.S. Consumer Product Safety Commission, 5401 Westbard Avenue, Room 625, Washington, DC 20207.
4. Specific information is available from the local chapter of the American Red Cross.
5. National Safety Town Center, P.O. Box 39312, Cleveland, OH 44139
6. National Safety Council, *Accident Facts, 1993 Edition* (Itasca, IL, 1993), 75.
7. Ibid., 74.

GLOSSARY

accident an occurrence that disrupts the flow of normal interactions and relationships which usually produces unintended injury, death, or property damage. (National Safety Council definition)

all-terrain vehicle (ATV) a motorized vehicle designed to travel on three or four low-pressure tires, capable of speeds of up to 40 miles per hour or more

amperes measurement of the flow of electricity

asphyxiation death resulting from carbon monoxide poisoning or the absence of oxygen

blizzard an abnormal amount of snow accompanied by high winds of at least 35 miles per hour

blood alcohol concentration (BAC) amount of alcohol in the bloodstream

burns tissue injuries usually caused by fire

caisson disease buildup of nitrogen in the bloodstream that occurs in scuba divers when they ascend too rapidly

center of gravity the center of mass of an object

combustion chemical process that causes a fire

corrosive substances substances that cause destruction of living tissue upon direct contact resulting from chemical action on the skin

deadman controls a mechanism which shuts off the auger and drive when the handle is released on a snow thrower

dram shop laws laws passed in several states which hold the providers of alcoholic beverages liable if they sell alcoholic beverages to an intoxicated person who later causes injury or death to a third person

fire chemical reaction in which rapid oxidation is combined with fuel

first collision the initial impact of the vehicle with another object

first-degree burn burn characterized by a reddening of the skin

flammability points points at which substances will burn

ground fault circuit interrupters (GFCIs) devices designed to shut off electricity when leakage of electric current is detected

hurricane a whirlwind of air that moves in a large spiral mass at winds of at least 75 miles per hour

hyperventilation disruption of normal respiration that occurs when there is prolonged deep and rapid breathing and a depression of carbon dioxide occurs

implied consent laws laws which require a driver to agree to a breath test whenever a law enforcement officer has reason to

289

believe that the individual is driving under the influence of alcohol

industrial hygienist individual that deals with environmental factors in the workplace that may cause sickness and injury

injury an unintentional or intentional damage to the body resulting from acute exposure to thermal, mechanical, electrical, or chemical energy or from the absence of such essentials as heat or oxygen. (National Committee for Injury Prevention and Control definition)

irritants noncorrosive substances that cause local inflammation of the skin upon prolonged or repeated contact

lightning a discharge of electricity that begins in a thundercloud

MADD acronym for Mothers Against Drunk Driving, a voluntary group interested in solving the problem of drunken driving

minibike a small, two-wheeled motorized cycle with a gasoline-driven engine about the size and power as that found on lawnmowers, capable of reaching speeds of 20 to 30 miles per hour

motorcycle a two-wheeled cycle which is operated by an engine with enough horsepower to run at speeds equivalent to motorized cars and trucks

National Electronic Injury Surveillance System a computerized clearinghouse that provides information about product-related injuries

occupational nurse a nurse who has specific training, experience, and skills unique to problems found in the workplace setting

occupational physician medical doctor who services the medical needs in the occupational setting

OSHA term used to identify the Occupational Safety and Health Administration

Richter scale unit of measurement used to record the strength of an earthquake

scald exposure to moist heat, hot water, and steam

scuba diving swimming about under water with a self-contained source of oxygen for breathing

second collision the collision that results from the forward momentum of the occupants in the motor vehicle after the first collision

second-degree burn burn which results in a deepened extent of damage to the skin, usually distinguished by the presence of blisters

sensitizers a substance to which an individual becomes allergic after exposure

skin diving swimming below the surface of the water while using a face mask, swimming fins, and snorkel. Sometimes referred to as snorkeling.

snowmobile a motorized vehicle which maneuvers on a pair of metal skis combined with a rubber belt tread

third-degree burn burn in which the entire layer of skin is affected

tornado a funnel cloud whirlwind, reaching 100 to 300 miles per hour, that forms along a front of warm, moist air and cool, dry air

tornado warning an alert that is issued when a tornado has been sighted

tornado watch an alert that is issued when conditions are present for a tornado to occur

toxic products agents which can produce personal injury or illness when ingested, inhaled, or absorbed through the skin

tunnel vision vision when the peripheral vision becomes impaired

volt current flowing through a wire moved by a force

watt the rate of using amperes of electricity pushed along by volts

wind chill the estimated temperature that is felt on the skin of an individual

CREDITS

Chapter 1
P. 7: © Bachman/Photri, Inc.; **p. 12:** AP/Wide World Photos; **p. 19:** © Dean Miller

Chapter 2
P. 39: Courtesy of The Reynolds Communications Group, Inc.; **p. 47:** © Gary Goodman/The Picture Cube; **p. 49:** © Owen Franken/Stock Boston; **p. 50:** Consumer Product Safety Commission; **p. 52:** © Spencer Grant/Monkmeyer Press

Chapter 3
P. 70: © Mark Antman/Stock Boston; **p. 72:** © L. Merrim/Monkmeyer Press

Chapter 4
P. 91: Reproduced with permission of Underwriters Laboratory, Inc.; **p. 94:** The Bettmann Archive

Chapter 5
P. 106: Occupational Safety and Health Administration; **p. 110 both:** National Institute for Occupational Safety and Health; **p. 114:** Occupational Safety and Health Administration; **p. 123:** AP/Wide World Photos

Chapter 6
P. 139: Courtesy Biology Systems Engineering, Institute of Agriculture and Natural Resources, University of Nebraska; **p. 141:** © Chromosohm Media/Stock Boston; **p. 148:** United States Department of Agriculture; **p. 149:** © Rob Crandall/Stock Boston

Chapter 7
P. 163 left: © Ken Robert Buck/The Picture Cube; **right:** Courtesy of Mothers Against Drunk Driving; **p. 174, 176:** Courtesy of The Chrysler Corporation; **p. 181:** Courtesy of Southern Pacific Lines/Joe Hanson Photography

Chapter 8
P. 191: © NOAA/Photri, Inc.; **p. 195:** National Hurricane Center/NOAA; **p. 202:** © Photri, Inc.; **p. 205:** © Kent Reno/Jeroboam; **p. 206:** © Spencer Grant/Monkmeyer Press

Chapter 9
P. 214: © Read D. Brugger/The Picture Cube; **p. 218:** © Audrey Gottlieb/Monkmeyer Press; **p. 225:** Courtesy of The Hunters Education Association and The Pennsylvania Game Commission

Chapter 10
P. 244, 248: Courtesy of The U.S. Coast Guard; **p. 252 left:** © Dean Miller; **right:** UPI/Bettmann

Chapter 11
P. 264: Courtesy of The Bureau of Community Services/Fire Safety Education/Photo by Fr. Jim Romeika; **p. 271:** © Katherine McGlynn/The Image Works, Inc.; **p. 276:** © Lora E. Askinazi/The Picture Cube; **p. 282:** © Dean Miller

INDEX

A, class fire, 83–84
A Safer Way For Everyday, 265
accident prone. *See* accident repetition
accident repetition, 10–13
accidents
    causation, 7–10
    term, 2–3, 5–6
active restraints. *See* seat belts
administrative license revocation, 165–66
aerosols, 66–67
Agriculture, U.S. Department of, 265
airbags, 175–77
alcohol, 86–87, 162–70, 240, 249–50
all-terrain vehicles (ATVs), 221–22
alternating current (AC), 45
American Academy of Pediatrics, 270
American Association of Poison Control Centers, 73
American Canoeing Association, 256
American College of Emergency Physicians, 272
American College of Surgeons, 272
American Red Cross, 255, 266
ammonia, 68, 146–47
amperes, 43
aspirin poisoning, 71
Association of Iron and Steel Electrical Engineers, 108
athletics, 281–83
ATV Specialty Vehicle Institute of America, 222
automatic sprinklers, 91

B, class fire, 84
back injuries, 119–20
bathroom, 35
blizzard, 199–201
blood-alcohol concentration (BAC), 162–63, 166, 249–50
blood-alcohol level, 162–63
boating, 243–50
booster cables, 160
buoys, 244
Bureau of Labor Statistics, 104, 110
bus driver, 273–74
bus maintenance, 274
bus routes, 275
bus transportation, school, 270–75

C, class fire, 84–85
caisson disease, 254
camping, 222–23
canoe, 250
carpal tunnel syndrome, 120
Census of Fatal Occupational Injuries, 104
Center for Environmental Health and Injury Control, 6, 74
chain saw, 39–40
chain saw kickback, 40
charcoal fires, 48
child restraints, 173–75
"childproof" matchbooks, 87
Christmas safety, 52–53
coal mining, 123–24
Coast Guard, United States, 243–44, 246, 248, 250

Coast Guard Auxiliary, 255
Commercial Driver's License Act, 125
community fire-fighting systems, 94
community pools, 242–43
compliance officer, OSHA, 113–14
Conference on Injury in America, 5–6
Consumer Product Safety Act, 59
Consumer Product Safety Commission, 35–36, 40, 51, 59–65, 70, 75, 76, 87, 221, 228, 231, 240–41, 255, 265–66
consumer safety, 57–76
correlation instruction, 262–63
cross-country skiing. *See* Nordic skiing
cumulative trauma disorders, 119–20
curriculum packages, 265–66
cycling, 227–30

D, class fire, 85
direct current (DC), 45
dram shop laws, 168
drowning, 239–40
drunk driving. *See* alcohol
dry pipe sprinkling system, 91–92

early fire warning systems, 90–92
earthquake, 203–7
educational reform, 261

293

electric mowers, 42
electrical shock. *See* electrocution
electricity, 43–46
electrocution, 148–49
emergency care, 275–78
emergency drills, 279–80
Emergency Medicine, 73
environmental factors, 10, 20
Environmental Protection Agency, 148
epidemiological model, 16–22
etiological agent, 19–20
extinguishing fires, 92–95

fabric flammability, 63–65
falls, 32–34
farm machinery, 137–43
Federal Coal Mine Health Act, 109
Federal Coal Mine Health and Safety Act, 124
Federal Hazardous Substances Act, 61, 65–66
Federal Highway Administration, 125
Federal Insecticide, Fungicide, and Rodenticide Act, 147
Federal Register, 111–12
fertilizers, 146
Field Sanitation Standard, 137
fire, 81–98, 143–44, 223, 247
fire, classifications, 83–85
firearms, 224–25
fireboats, 94
firecrackers, 50
fire drills, 279–80
fire engine, 94
fire-fighting personnel, 95
fireplace, 37–38
fire prevention, 95–96
Fire Prevention Week, 264–65
fire safety ladders, 96
fireworks, 50–51
first collision, 170–71
First Cooperative Safety Congress, 108
first-degree burn, 88
flame detectors, 91
Flammable Fabrics Act, 61, 63
flammable liquids, 46–48
flashflood, 202–3
floods, 201–3
food poisoning, 69

forestry, 149–50
4-H Clubs, 136, 143
Future Farmers of America (FFA), 136, 143

gasoline, 47–48
GFCI. *See* ground fault circuit interrupters
grain storage, 143–45
ground fault circuit interrupters, 44

Halloween, 51–52
Hazard Communication Standard, 137
heat sensory detector, 91
helmets, 217–18, 221, 229–30
Highway Safety Act, 272
hip fracture, 32
history, occupational safety, 105–9
holiday safety, 50–51
home fire escape plan, 97–98
home pools, 241–42
home safety, 29–53
  children, 30–31
  elderly, 31–32
home workshops, 38–39
host, 18–19
human factors, 7–9
hunting, 223–25
hurricane, 193–97
Hurricane Andrew, 195–97
Hurricane Hugo, 194–96
Hurricane Iniki, 195–96
hyperventilation, 254

ice safety, 250–52
Illinois chapter, American Academy of Pediatrics, 73
Illinois Steel Company, 107
imminent danger, 112
impact restraints, 171–78
implied consent laws, 166–67, 250
incidental instruction, 261–62
industrial hygienist, 121
injury, definition, 6
injury, relating to fire, 87–90
inspection priorities, 112–13
inspections, occupational safety, 112–14
interlock system, 172

ion chamber detector, 91
It's No Accident, 266

jellyfish, 254

kitchen, 34–35

labeling, products, 65
Labor, U.S. Department of, 108–9
lawnmowers, 41–42
legal drinking age, 167–68
licensure, 218–19, 244
life jackets. *See* personal flotation devices
lightning, 197–99
liquid poisons, 69
"locking-on" effect, 45

MADD. *See* Mothers Against Drunk Driving
manure waste pit, 145–46
marine animals, 254–55
marine radio, 245
mechanical factors, 9–10
medical procedures, burns, 89–90
medications, 68–69
methane, 146
Mine Safety and Health Administration, 124
minibike, 219–20
mining, 122–24
Mining Enforcement Safety and Health Administration, 124
mobile homes, 48–50, 192–93, 196
monetary awards, 14–15
Mothers Against Drunk Driving, 163, 166
motor vehicle crashes
  age factors, 159
  environmental factors, 160–62
  human factors, 158–59
  vehicular factors, 159–60
motor vehicle safety, 155–81
motorcycle, 216–19
motorcycle burn, 217
Motorcycle Safety Foundation, 219
motorized recreational vehicles, 213–22

National Athletic Trainers Association, 284–85
National Coalition for Seat Belts in School Buses, 272
National Council for Industrial Safety, 108
National Electronic Injury Surveillance System (NEISS), 60, 62
National Farm Safety Week, 265
National Fire Protection Association, 37, 95–96, 107, 264
national health objectives, 22–23, 32–33, 86, 90, 119–20, 158, 162, 173, 218, 239
National Highway Traffic Safety Administration, 160, 166, 174, 216, 272
National Injury Control Conference, 88
National Institute for Occupational Safety and Health (NIOSH), 109
National Poison Prevention Week, 72
National Recreation and Parks Association, 270
National Research Council, National Academy of Science, 5
National Rifle Association, 225
National Safety Council, 104–5, 108, 139, 166, 219, 265, 278
National School Transportation Association, 273
National Ski Patrol, 226
National Spa and Pool Institute, 255
National Transportation Safety Administration, 273
National Transportation Safety Board report, 273
National Weather Service, U.S., 196, 199
NEISS. *See* National Electronic Injury Surveillance System (NEISS)
NEISS News, 62
Nordic skiing, 227

occupational nurse, 121–22
occupational physician, 121–22
occupational safety, 103–27

Occupational Safety and Health Act (1970), 109–19, 122, 126
Occupational Safety and Health Administration (OSHA), 109, 111–14, 116–19, 136–37, 145
occupational skin disorders, 120
Operation Water Watch, 255

passive restraints, 175–78
pedestrian safety, 179–80
penalties, 114
personal flotation devices, 246–47
personal protective equipment, 126
pesticides, 146–48
photoelectric detector, 90–91
physiology of alcohol, 162–64
playground, school, 270
poison control centers, 73
Poison Prevention Packaging Act, 61, 70–71
poisoning, 67–73
polyvinyl chloride (PVC), 89
portable fire extinguisher, 93
Power Squadron, U.S., 255
power takeoff shaft (PTO), 138
preschool safety instruction, 267
product recall, 159–60
public playgrounds, 231–32

railroad crossing, 180–81
reaction time, 164
rear overturn, 140
recreation, 211–32
Refrigerator Safety Act, 61
rescue equipment, water, 243
research, occupational safety, 111
Richter scale, 204
rights and responsibilities, occupational safety, 115
rollover protective structures (ROPS), 141–42
rural safety, 133–50

safe school environment, 268–70
safety, definition, 5
safety engineering, 16
safety engineers, 121
safety instruction, 261–68
safety motivational programs, 126–27

Safety Town Program, 267
sailboat, 250
San Andreas Fault, 204
scalding, 88
school accident records, 278
school safety, 259–85
scuba diving, 253–54
seat belts, 142, 171–75, 272
second collision, 170–71
second-degree burn, 88
secondary enforcement, 173
side overturn, 140
silo entrapment, 144–45
ski boots, 226
skiing, 225–27
skin diving, 253
smoke detector, 90
smoking, 87
snorkeling. *See* skin diving
snow throwers, 42
snowmobile, 213–15
sobriety checkpoints, 167
Social Security Administration, 108
speed limit, 178
standards, occupational safety, 111
state OSHA, 116
stop-drop-roll, 97, 263
supervision, athletics, 283
Surface Transportation and Uniform Relocation Act, 178–79
surfing, 252
Surgeon General's Workshop on Drunk Driving, 169–70

television, 36–37
third-degree burn, 88
Third National Injury Control Conference, 74
third-party responsibility, 168–69
three-pronged plugs, 44
tornado, 190–93
tornado drills, school, 280
tornado warning, 192
tornado warning drill, school, 193
tornado watch, 192
toxic gases, 145–46
toy safety, 74–76, 228
tractors, 139–43
transportation, 125
Transportation, U.S. Department of, 125, 168, 177

tsunami, 203
"tunnel vision," 163–64
typhoon, 194

Underwriter Laboratory (UL), 53, 107
Uniform Minimum Drinking Age Act, 198

ventilation, grain storage, 145
violations, 113–14
vocational education, 262

Walsh-Healey Acts, 108–9
water instruction, 255–56

water safety, 237–56
water skiing, 255
water slides, 242–43
watts, 43
wet pipe sprinkler system, 91–92
wind chill factor, 200–201
worker's compensation, 107–8